RADIOLOGY MANAGEMENT

A GUIDE FOR ADMINISTRATORS, SUPERVISORS, AND STUDENTS

VOLUME 2

Eric Bouchard

SHEPHERD INC

10340 MILITARY RD · P.O. BOX 1861
DUBUQUE · IOWA · 52004-1861

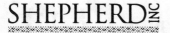
ISBN Volume 1 1-881795-04-7
      Volume 2 1-881795-05-5
      Set   1-881795-06-3

Manufactured in the United States of America.

10 9 8 7 6 5 4 3 2 1

*This book is lovingly dedicated
to my daughters, Erin and Lauren.*

CONTENTS

Preface   vii
Acknowledgments   ix
About the Author   xi
Introduction   xiii

VOLUME I

SECTION ONE PEOPLE   1

1.1   Radiologic Administration: Structure and Style   2
1.2   The Manpower Shortage in Radiologic Technologies   14
1.3   Job Descriptions   17
1.4   Selecting Personnel   36
1.5   Orienting the New Employee   47
1.6   Measuring Performance   56
1.7   Counseling the Ineffective Employee   62
1.8   Clinical Ladders   68
1.9   Managing Productivity   77
1.10 Recruiting and Retaining Professional Staff   84
1.11 Promoting Your Own Career   94
1.12 Customer Relations   100
1.13 Customer Relations Training   103
1.14 Communicating with Medical Staff   108

SECTION TWO TECHNOLOGY   113

2.1   Radiology Information Systems   114
2.2   Picture Archiving and Communication Systems   127
2.3   Writing Equipment Specifications   138
2.4   Mobile Technology   148
2.5   Positron Emission Tomography   154
2.6   Lasers in Medicine   167
2.7   The Business of Mammography   170
2.8   Technology Assessment   182
2.9   Future Trends in Technology   188
2.10 Financing New Technology   200

v

2.11 MRI—Feasibility of A New Service   204
2.12 MRI Purchase Considerations   212
2.13 OSHA Safety Requirements for Hazardous
      Chemicals in the Workplace   216

List of References   227
Index   245

VOLUME II

SECTION THREE PLANNING   1

3.1 Certificate of Need   2
3.2 Writing a Business Plan   7
3.3 Working with Consultants   12
3.4 Marketing Imaging Services   14
3.5 Directory of Radiologic Organizations   35
3.6 Policies and Procedures   59
3.7 Strategic Planning   68
3.8 Facility Planning   80

SECTION FOUR MANAGING   117

4.1   Service Line Management   118
4.2   The New Manager   120
4.3   Total Quality Management   124
4.4   Radiology Benchmarking   138
4.5   Cost Containment   143
4.6   Licensure of Radiologic Professionals   149
4.7   Joint Ventures   152
4.8   The Joint Commission on Accreditation of
      Healthcare Organizations   159
4.9   Risk Management and Liability Prevention   187
4.10 Basic Healthcare Financial Management   208
4.11 Quality-Assessment and Improvement   244

List of References   267
Index   285

Preface

In 1983, my first book titled *Radiology Management: An Introduction* was published. It was my belief that students and new radiology managers wanted a straightforward, practically-oriented text to use as a guide to the daily operations of a radiology department. The book had a wide appeal to instructors, students, and practicing managers. Nearly nine years later, I met radiology managers who said they were still using that book!

Obviously, the point had been reached where further development and refinement of the useful information found in the first book was necessary. The dynamic changes in radiology management over the last decade required that alteration, deletion, and expansion of previously-presented material be made.

The result was a new book, *Radiology Manager's Handbook*. When it was in final preparation in the spring of 1992, Mary Jess of Shepherd, Inc. called to say...."You need to find a stopping place, this book won't fit in a one inch binding!" So I stopped sending material to the publisher but I didn't stop writing and collecting my radiology management "pearls."

In this second edition, the string of pearls gets longer with over 50 separate new illustrations and chapter sections or appendices. Don't think of this updated version, *Radiology Management: A Guide for Administrators, Supervisors, and Students Vol. 1 and 2* as strictly new editions but as additions to my attempt to bring a concise yet comprehensive desk reference to the busy radiology manager.

The purpose of this handbook is to introduce the reader to a subject area and offer useful examples easily adapted for use in today's radiology department.

It is my hope that this handbook will stimulate further interest in radiology management as a field of study. I believe that radiology management is a dynamic and changing field and that this text offers practical, useful applications in the "real world" of radiology management.

Eric Bouchard
July 1993

Acknowledgments

Thanks to Michael Stephen Kuber again for his permission to reprint "Radiology Administration: Structure and Style." Thanks to Mary Louise Wright for her permission to reprint information on radiology reimbursement and to Sandra Harrison for her help with career ladders. The American College of Radiology has been very gracious in allowing me to use material on contract media management, reporting and mammography. Rick Martinez of *Administrative Radiology Magazine* allowed many uses and citations, and Peter J. Bartolazzi contributed valuable information on equipment specifications. Credit also goes to Jim Dohms of Sarasota, Florida for the chapter he contributed on hazardous materials, the RMBA for coding and nomenclature for stereotactic breast biopsy, *Second Source Imaging Magazine* for an extensive figure describing the current state of bone densitometry and the department of nursing at Baptist Hospital of East Tennessee for assistance with the career ladder discussion.

Blaine Lester of Johnstown, Pennsylvania contributed two figures for employee selection, and the directory of technologist education in MRI originally appeared in *RT Image Magazine*. Alan Weinstein contributed the new chapter on Radiology Benchmarking and Monica Langley of Knoxville, Tennessee helped with ADA as it relates to hiring. I am also grateful to Anthony G. Lyon, M.D., for his encouragement, and I am deeply appreciative of the numerous sources of adapted material in this text. Finally, I need to mention that the inspiration for this project comes from my long time association with the American Healthcare Radiology Administrators.

Special thanks to Pat Eichhorst at Shepherd for expert editing, careful proofreading and attention to all those last minute details.

Eric Bouchard, FAHRA

About the Author

Eric Bouchard, B.S., M.A., R.T. (R) is the Director-Center for NeuroSciences and Rehabilitation at Baptist Hospital of East Tennessee, Knoxville, Tennessee. He is also a Fellow of the American Healthcare Radiology Administrators and has previously published both books and articles on the subject of radiology management.

INTRODUCTION

This book on the subject of radiology management is a compilation of information on topics relevant to anyone interested in radiology management. The book is organized under four major sections with subheadings listing subjects often unique to the field of radiology management. As the field of radiology management has grown sophisticated, so have the information needs of radiology managers and students. Today's busy radiology departments have leadership at numerous supervisory levels. These levels of expertise have a knowledge of radiology management that is varied. What is particularly attractive about a handbook-style treatment of this subject is quick reference. Instructors also find this format useful since each section can stand alone and information can be gleaned from selected areas. In particular, practical lessons and examples that the radiology manager may adapt are prominent aspects of this handbook.

The content of this book is a straightforward treatment of subjects specific and unique to radiology management. No attempt is made to present a topic in its entirety; rather, radiology managers will find the concise approach to various subjects a very attractive feature of the book. As much as possible, subjects included in this handbook are on the cutting edge of radiology management.

The material is organized under the administrative functions of people, technology, planning, and management. The length of each of the 46 sections varies depending upon the difficulty of the subject. The book contains charts, graphs, and examples. A major characteristic of this handbook is the use of descriptive materials.

The most distinguishing feature of this book is the way in which the material is organized. This is the only handbook-style treatment of the subject of radiology management published today. This quick reference-style text will benefit the reader because of the ease with which information about a specific subject can be found. This book is an indispensable reference for managers at all levels and students too.

The author

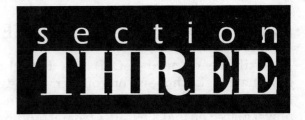

PLANNING

3.1   CERTIFICATE OF NEED

3.2   WRITING A BUSINESS PLAN

3.3   WORKING WITH CONSULTANTS

3.4   MARKETING IMAGING SERVICES

3.5   DIRECTORY OF RADIOLOGIC ORGANIZATIONS

3.6   POLICIES AND PROCEDURES

3.7   STRATEGIC PLANNING

3.8   FACILITY PLANNING

3.1 CERTIFICATE OF NEED

Certificate of need (CON) was thought to be the federal government's last hope of controlling rising healthcare costs. In 1974, it began as a national health-planning program. Today the amount of power placed on the CON, after federal funding ended in 1986, is up to individual states. Less than 30 states have retained a CON process; some of these states have CON rules stringent enough to impact the acquisition of imaging equipment. See figure 3.1 for a sampling of CON state programs.The diversity in CON rules from state to state is amazing. In addition to thresholds on capital acquisitions and improvements, there are numerous exemptions in individual state laws for types of equipment, ownership arrangements, and service volumes.

Understanding the Health-Planning Process

When health planning comes to mind, visions of what is practical, economical, and positive are most prominent. While it is agreed that health planning is a rational concept, wide disagreement exists concerning the methods of planning.

The duties of the radiology department administrator are affected by government regulation. Public views about healthcare delivery largely depend on images imposed by the news media and by personal experience with health costs, which are rising at an alarming rate. The need for closer controls on healthcare delivery is a foregone conclusion. Hospital management must accept these controls and use them to their most productive ends.

The burden of regulating healthcare costs has been passed on to the consumer. The National Health Planning and Resources Development Act of 1974 provided consumers with the power to regulate healthcare through local health systems agencies. The intent of the law was to plan for healthcare, resources, and services that were equal in access and reasonable in cost to the entire community.

Figure 3.1 The status of state CON programs and initiatives changes constantly, but most legislation under consideration is clearly intended to increase state control of healthcare delivery.

CON and Other Regulations for Major Medical Equipment

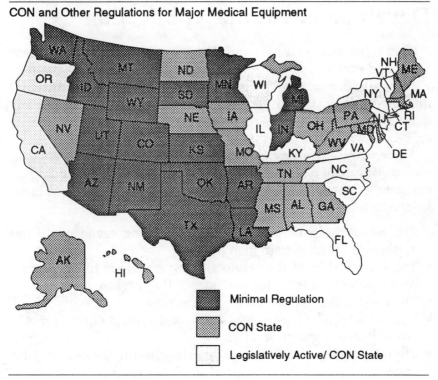

Adapted from Kyes, Kris. A Nationwide Review. *Decisions in Imaging Economics*. Vol. 5, No. 3, 1992.

Certificate of Need Process

The most important area of interface for the radiology manager is the project review or certificate of need process. The following is a step-by-step synopsis of the certificate of need procedure. It should be noted that this process will vary from state to state.

Determination of Reviewabilty

The CON staff should be contacted to explain the scope of the project and the estimated cost. A determination will be made of whether the project needs to be reviewed based on state regulations applicable in the area.

Development of the Application

This is the most complex and detailed step. First, the necessary forms and review manual from the CON office should be obtained. This manual outlines the information needed in the application and the standards by which the project is reviewed. If there are any questions or uncertainties, a predevelopment conference can be requested with the CON staff.

There are nine primary areas of concern that must be addressed in each certificate of need application. These areas vary depending on the state, but the basic content of the application addresses these following areas:

- The relationship of the health service being reviewed to the applicable health system plan (HSP).
- The relationship of the services being reviewed to long-range development plans for the provider of the services.
- The need of the population for such services.
- The availability of alternatives — less costly, more effective methods of providing such services.
- The relationship of services to the existing healthcare system of the area.
- The availability of resources, including health staffing management personnel and funds for capital and operating to provide such services, and the availability of alternative uses of such resources to provide other health services.
- The special need and circumstances of the healthcare providers who supply a substantial portion of services and resources to individuals not residing in their healthcare area, such as: medical schools, multidisciplinary clinics, and specialty centers.
- The special needs and circumstances of health maintenance organizations.

- The special needs when a construction project is required to implement such services; the costs, methods, and impact of the construction project would be reviewed.

Review for Completeness

The CON staff reviews the application submitted and requests additional information as necessary. A specified time frame is given during which the additional information requested can be collected.

Solicitation of Public Comments

Once the application is determined to be complete, the CON staff solicits public comments. The culmination of the public comment phase is the holding of a public hearing prior to the CON decision on the application.

Review by the CON Staff

The CON staff reviews the application. Normally, representatives from the facilities submitting the application are invited to respond to questions by the CON staff.

Appeal Process

Every state must have an approved appeal process for applications that are denied. The CON review manual should specify the appeal process.

The certificate of need process is a well-defined procedure that involves a lengthy application phase and time for clear thinking and writing. This is the initial step toward any purchase of a major piece of equipment or implementation of a new service. The typical review process takes from 90 to 120 days.

Figure 3.2 Utilization Section of a Typical Certificate of Need Application

---

Department Utilization

1. How many patients referred to your institution had medical problems or diseases for which this new expanded service could be appropriately used?
   Inpatient _____   Outpatient _____

2. How many radiographic procedures were conducted in the last calendar year?
   _____

3. What change in volume do you anticipate after installation of equipment?
   Present volume _____
   1st year after installation +_____-_____
   2nd year after installation +_____-_____

4. What change in man hours do you anticipate after installation of equipment?
   Present volume _____
   1st year after installation +_____-_____
   2nd year after installation +_____-_____

5. If man hours are increased how many full time equivalents will be added to the departmental budget? _____
   What will be the average yearly salary paid to these employees?
   _____

6. What change in patient days do you anticipate after installation of equipment?
   Present patient days _____
   1st year patient days +_____-_____
   2nd year patient days +_____-_____

Lille, K. "Applying for a Certificate of Need." *Radiology/Nuclear Medicine Magazine.* 7(4):29, 1977.

Conclusion

Figure 3.2 is an example of a typical utilization review section as it may appear in certificate of need applications. In supplying information about utilization, it is important to understand that the CON staff will critically look at the need for the project. The radiology manager should be familiar with local and state health-planning regulations in order to write proposals for the improvement or expansion of radiology services. The U.S. healthcare system is criticized for spiraling costs, poor distribution of services, and ineffective healthcare practices, resulting in criticism that has prompted health-planning policy. The certificate of need process is well defined in intent, and while time consuming, is not an impenetrable fortress of government bureaucracy.

3.2 WRITING A BUSINESS PLAN

The Business Plan Is a Key Management Tool

A business plan is a formal document that becomes the operational blueprint for a proposed new activity. It gives your program a sense of direction and a focus for future development. The quality of your plan will be a major factor in determining whether the new activity is worthy of funding. The business plan is also a management tool. It will help you focus in a logical and organized fashion on the future growth of your enterprise. It will help to anticipate and meet the challenges of a changing environment, and it functions as a control tool—a set of checks and balances that allow you to monitor and assess program successes.

Components of the Business Plan

A business plan could consist of up to ten major components. Some components are optional depending upon the special needs of your project and the purpose for writing the plan. The list of components described here is just a framework in order to uniquely tailor your plan. Your plan should ultimately fit your organization's specific needs and characteristics.

Executive Summary

Although the plan summary appears first, it is the last to be written. Your goal in the summary is to quickly and concisely provide the reader with an overview. The ideal executive summary will be three to five pages long. A very short business plan may not need a summary section; however, if your plan exceeds ten pages then the summary is essential. The plan summary will highlight key elements of the entire business plan, including:

- Objective for the project.
- Description of products and services.

- Market potential and competition.
- Projected financial outcomes.
- Capital needs and return on investment.

Background and History

When you work for a company that has a long history, a summary of past accomplishments and highlights of specific successes belong in this section. Also, if your organization has undergone significant changes in philosophy, you may wish to include a brief description of how these changes in mission came about. This section is the appropriate place to draw comparisons of similar efforts and the reasons for their failures or successes. This is an opportunity to expound on your uniqueness and potential for success where others have floundered. You could discuss strategies for service delivery, previously untapped markets, and new locations. Or, you may wish to save discussion of these aspects of the market and competition for later in the plan. Describe your background and history adequately. Focus your plan on the present and the future.

The Product

The programs and services you provide flow directly from the mission statement. The mission statement will be the first item in this section. Following the mission statement describe the purpose, goals, and objectives that will lead to the completion of your stated goals. This is the most important section of the business plan. It will distinquish your products or services from all others, and support any assertions you make about how your project will be a success. This section can include the following information:

- Description of the product—Describe the key features of your product or service and its benefits to potential customers.
- Proprietary position—Tell about a copyright or patent position you may have. How will you gain a superior position in your industry?
- Special arrangements—Detail conditions that will discourage competition. Describe exclusive arrangements with dealers or innovations in service delivery.

- Product extension—New product development to reflect the expected changing market needs and to protect the long term viability of the company would be detailed here. Also, research and development activities on current products as well as future products need to be stated in layman's terms.

The Market Analysis

Here is where you show how the idea for a product or service turns into something of consumer interest. In this section you will need to build a case for the entry of your product into the market place. You will need to convince the reader of the following major points:

1. That there is a need for your product.
2. That you understand that need and how your product will satisfy it.
3. That you can sell it for a profit.

The Competition

The purpose of this section of the plan is to demonstrate your understanding of the competition, what their constituency is, and how their activities may affect yours. Competition can actually compliment your program by describing the differences in perspective customers, geography, and programmatic details, emphasizing the unique qualities of your proposed project. You will need to discuss the major potential customers you plan to attract by responding to questions such as:

1. Who will be your customer?
2. Why will they buy from you?
3. When will they buy?
4. What are the expectations of the customer for service, price, and quality?
5. What is the market share of your competition?
6. How will your service be different from others?
7. What are your competitors' strengths and weaknesses?

Marketing Plans

Marketing activities are supposed to attract a specific audience for your product or service. Your marketing plan will attend to the general image you are trying to project and how you will advertise your products or services. A specific goal of the marketing plan will be to describe the methodology you will use to document public awareness of your program. This section of the plan will demonstrate that you understand your market and that you have the ability to sell to a targeted audience. This is where you show why customers will choose to buy from you. Describe in some detail:

1. Your understanding of how to segment and target your market.
2. Your estimate of sales and market share projected up to five years.
3. Your pricing plan and how it allows you to be competitive and make a profit.
4. Your sales plan describing your sales efficiency and method of distribution.
5. Your promotional plan detailing how you will generate awareness of your products and services to potential customers.

Financial Information

The financial section of your business plan will be more closely scrutinized than any other information you submit. It will identify the amount of money needed to support operations and the amount of revenues necessary to offset expenses and product profits. Typically, there will be financial assumptions, a three or five year proforma, and a prediction of revenue sources. The basic assumptions such as expected volumes, growth predictions, and contractual adjustments should be made in financial terms and be as realistic as possible. Financial projections will include operating expenses, capital expenses, interest expenses, and revenues. The financial section of your business plan will have at least the following exhibits:

A. Projected statement of operations.
B. Cash flow.
C. Proforma.
D. Break even analysis.

A final note of consideration about financial disclosures (since this material is often sensitive and very confidential): plan to control distribution of your business plan carefully.

Organizational Structure

This is where you will find the organizational chart. The organizational chart depicts who's who in your management structure and should include the number of persons and the types of positions they hold. You can also describe the kind of governance your organization will have. The composition of the board, its purpose, and its involvement in operations can be outlined here. Appended to this section are usually brief biographies of key management and a list of board members with their affiliations.

Evaluation

Measuring success will differ from one organization to another. In your program plan pay particular attention to developing evaluation tools that will be consistent over time. One of the major reasons for writing a business plan is to demonstrate why you will have a successful venture. Your evaluation tools should flow from goals and objectives you articulated earlier in the plan. It is essential that the data you use for measurement be easily collectible and helpful in drawing meaningful conclusions. Be careful not to get overwhelmed with collecting too much information. Rather, find ten or so success measures that will allow you to monitor your program's effectiveness at accomplishing its mission.

Final Hints

Your business plan should not exceed 50 pages in length. You don't want to smother a great idea by turning off the reader with needless jargon. Make it easy for the reader to find the information desired by providing a good table of contents. Lastly, pay attention to the appearance of your finished plan. A good presentation conveys to the reader that you have taken a professional approach and consider the work you propose to be a serious matter.

3.3 WORKING WITH CONSULTANTS

Consultants have become commonplace in healthcare. Finding the best consultant to meet the hospital's needs for the dollars that you can afford is not an easy task. What makes a good consultant and how do you go about finding one?

When faced with projects that need to be completed, hospital management must consider whether time and talent in the organization is available to accomplish the needed planning and activation. Hospital managers today are increasingly more specialized due to the enormous technical sophistication of healthcare delivery. Managers therefore cannot be expected to know everything about a burgeoning technical discipline. Sometimes outside help is necessary. Once the decision is made to hire a consultant, a list of potential candidates can be developed using personal recommendations, referrals from professional organizations, directories of specific kinds of consultant firms, and possibly the faculty of a local university. The candidates would then submit proposals to do the work based on their understanding of the scope and nature of the project.

A proposal to provide consultative services should include at least the following items:

- Background information on the consulting firm.
- The approach to the management problem.
- The method used to provide documentation.
- Understanding of the field and experience with similar projects.
- Experience and qualifications of the consultants.
- Detailed costs of services.
- Estimated travel expenses and per diems.
- Other client references (See Figure 3.3).
- Project completion time frame.
- Hospital and consultant responsibilities.

Why Use Outside Talent?

Using an outside consultant with industry knowledge and the expected ability to produce quick results is often the chief reason for the decision to call an expert. Usually, it takes less time to launch a new program this way. In addition, consultants bring great access to

Figure 3.3 Checking Consultant References

- Overall satisfaction with engagement.
- Quality of interaction with hospital staff.
- Timeliness of reports.
- Problem identification and solutions suggested.
- Any weaknesses in overall approach.
- Did consultants meet objectives set forth in the proposal?
- Was the fee structure reasonable for services received?
- Would consultants be used again?

data and are generally more creative and unbiased in approaches to problems. It can also be much less costly to use a consultant for a quick start-up of a potentially large revenue producing venture. In cost reduction strategies where consultants are used extensively, immediate cost savings can offset the expenses associated with consultative services.

Using In-House Talent

Before deciding to use a consultant, review your in-house resources to determine whether you have the expertise already on board to attack the problem. Possibly, there is a talented individual on staff who could be trained to do the job at minimal expense. Also, consider hiring a full-time employee to accomplish the task with a plan to continually utilize this person for other projects. There are pitfalls in doing an in-house project. Often the individual assigned to the project has other duties or needs a period of learning before actual project work proceeds. Bias can cloud the success of a project as well. Outside experts tend to have more success at "selling" new concepts. The in-house talent rarely enjoys the halo of expertise that the outside talent is assumed to possess. Lastly, because healthcare managers have become increasingly more specialized, it is difficult to find in-house talent with the broad based ability to be knowledgeable in state-of-the-art practices in all parts of the hospital.

Choosing the Consultant

Look for a firm with an objective, straight forward approach to doing business, a proven results-oriented track record, and good client references. Investigate to see that the firm is fiscally sound and the consulting staff is knowledgeable in the subject areas you need probed. Although price is a major consideration, the key determinant when choosing a consultant is expertise. Use the following to assist you in choosing the best consultant for your hospital's needs:

1. Only consider consultants with healthcare experience.
2. Look for firms specializing in your particular area of interest.
3. Match the capabilities of the firm with your specific needs.
4. Use a request for proposal process.
5. Know who your consultant(s) will be.
6. Compare firms on the basis of how they will accomplish the work, not just on the price.

3.4   MARKETING IMAGING SERVICES

Advanced medical equipment, such as that found in the modern full-service radiology department, is a strategic tool that will attract both physician referrals and patient inquiries. High technology equipment is getting more marketing attention now that the provider environment is so competitive; hospitals are maximizing opportunities to get a return on these high-dollar investments. The high price of technology for hospitals places a great economic pressure on these providers to recoup acquisition costs.

Communication with physicians and patients is critical to successfully marketing technology. Experts agree that education is the key; that is, informing physicians and the public about new high technology options available and about the capabilities of this new equipment. Public promotion can make a marketing difference with services where the patient has some influence over the selection of the provider.

One hospital used a public promotion campaign to promote a new color flow untrasound machine that it had acquired. It mailed 25,000 flyers to households in its service area that described the new diagnostic capabilities of the machine. The direct-mail campaign was supplemented with billboard advertising that featured the hospital as a technological leader in the community. Additional ultrasound volume resulted from the campaign, and hospital market share of ultrasound studies was stabilized. A dwindling of market share that had been occuring due to private office competition was averted.

Consider this story of a retired businessman in Jacksonville, Florida, who won a PET scan at a charity auction. It was by no accident that this PET scan was offered as a sale item. The scan was just a piece of a marketing strategy by a local hospital to increase consumer awareness of this new high technology service. By coincidence this businessman had attended a local Rotary Club meeting and heard a presentation on PET by a cardiologist affiliated with the local hospital that donated the PET scan to the charity auction. The businessman later bid on the PET scan because he had become an informed consumer; the cardiologist's lecture had influenced this decision. The PET scan revealed a potentially life-threatening block in a coronary artery and resulted in the need for balloon angioplasty. Of course, the hospital charged for the additional studies, which is business they might not have received if not for these simple PET marketing efforts.

High technology capability and outstanding image quality alone will not assure that utilization will meet proforma predictions as outlined in your business plan. Attention to every detail is necessary to establish a reputation as a provider with the best value. A major attribute that contributes to the perception of quality service is waiting times; for patients, it's exam turnaround time; for physicians, it's timely receipt of the report. At a Florida hospital, report turnaround time has improved with a facsimile machine connected to the hospital's results reporting computer system. The hospital states that a hard copy of the report via FAX is transmitted to the referring physician within four hours after the exam is completed. Dr. Elias Zerhouni of Johns Hopkins Hospital in Baltimore instituted a sophisticated FAX network to referring physicians when he discovered it took up to ten days for his MRI reports to be delivered. Since the hospital began using the FAX method of report transmission, exam volume in MRI has nearly doubled. The marketing lesson was determining the expectations of referring physicians and tailoring the service to meet those expectations.

At a multimodality imaging center in New York City, a marketing representative visits every physician following a first time referral. The center also publishes a periodic promotional letter that uses case histories and images to show the diagnosis. Another center in Wisconsin uses a referral kit for the referring physician's office staff. For the physician a special reference guide to MRI indicators is distributed and updated periodically. A center in Spokane, Washington, reports success with sponsoring physician educational programs with CME credit. They use focus group style information by gathering at informal luncheons with office managers of their referring physicians. At these sessions they learn about how their services are perceived by their users and what the patients tell their physicians about the imaging services that they have received.

Marketing Perspective

The Narrow View

Marketing is viewed and implemented too narrowly by physicians and administrators. The Narrow View is the first most frequent mistake made about marketing. Marketing is recognizing the multiple constituencies available and exercising the full range of strategies and tactics to attract the customer. These multiple constituencies include the physician, patient, employers, third-party payers, the government, health-related agencies, and employees. Marketing is not just advertising and promotion; it is a comprehensive process of selling in any number of skillful combinations. Marketing is a deliberate endeavor to build business in an informed and carefully calculated manner. The components of a comprehensive marketing program are as follows:

1. **Research and Analysis:** Market research and analysis strengthens the marketing plan by expanding your knowledge base of a referral area.

    General Electric Medical Systems has software that analyzes demographics and projected demand for imaging services in any geographic area. Their programs can analyze projected patient volume and pricing, and can compare changes in competing technology and how those changes could affect current modalities. This demographic mapping software gives the radiology department a "crystal ball" to predict how imaging services will perform in the future.

Analysis of customer needs assures that services are available to benefit the customer. Patient surveys, understanding the demographics of your service area, and identifying trends are some parts of market research. Figure 3.4 describes some negative and positive aspects of information gathering using personal interviews, telephone interviews, and mailed surveys. Also see chapter appendix A for more views on information gathering.

Figure 3.4

Some views on methods used to gather consumer information.

Personal Interviews
Positive Aspects:
• Allows interviewer to probe for detailed information
• Allows interviewer to build relationships with potential patients
Negative Aspects:
• Interviewers must be recruited, screened, and trained.
• Process is time-consuming
• Cost may be high due to time involved.
• Objectivity may be reduced.

Telephone Interviews
Positive Aspects:
• Allows interviewer to probe for detailed information
• Cost in time and money is lower than for personal interviews.
• Process is more expedient and should be used when time is critical.
Negative Aspects:
• The telephone survey is more costly than a mail survey.
• Respondents may terminate the call.
• Interviewers must be trained to ask for details, to be objective and not lead responses, and to complete the survey.

Mailed Surveys
Positive Aspects:
• Mailed surveys are inexpensive.
• Mailed surveys can allow for respondent anonymity.
• Mailed surveys prevent interviewer bias.
• Mailed surveys allow respondents to be more truthful about sensitive issues.
Negative Aspects:
• Response rates are low. Sample may be too low for analysis.
• Mailed surveys offer no opportunity to probe.
• Anonymity prevents reaching the respondent for follow-up.
• Mailed surveys provide no opportunity to foster relationships.

Adapted from Leiter, P. and Jacobson, S.L. "Sound Marketing for Offsite Private Practices." *Rehab Management* 4:6,1990.

2. **Strategic Planning:** Prioritizing the practice opportunities and the tactics needed to attract the business are strategically planned. Once a target market is identified with the assistance of market research, then a plan to attract that market is implemented. Examples of tactics that might be in place to meet the general goals of the marketing plan would be:

    - Promote community awareness of the imaging services.
    - Distinguish these services from all others with a unique selling point.
    - Develop new imaging applications.
    - Recruit new referring physicians.
    - Develop a plan for encouraging repeat referrals.

3. **Product Development:** Identifying new services for a market and modifying existing services to changing technology are the tasks of product development in medical imaging. Again, the data collected in market research and analysis guides the decisions about new services. With each new service capability, the need for planning the introduction of that service to the community occurs again. Your products and services should be assessed on a periodic basis to determine if you continue to meet current market demand and whether you are capitalizing on opportunities to penetrate new markets. The following list will assist you in auditing your product/service profile.

    - List your organization's products and services, both present and proposed.
    - Describe the outstanding characteristics of each product or service.
    - What distinctiveness of services sets you apart from your competitors?
    - Look at the charges for your services. Are the charges in line with the market?
    - What services are used the most? Why?
    - Who are the users of your services? Are they divided into distinct groups?
    - What are the most common complaints against the services provided?

4. **Pricing:** Establishing a price structure for your services is influenced by your costs, but the true barometer of your price making strategy is market-based input. Pricing has become the most important element in the entire marketing process because of the active roles of business and insurers to control healthcare costs. Evaluate your pricing practices by researching the answers to these questions:

   - What is the pricing methodology for your organization?
     —Cost plus.
     —Return on investment (ROI).
     —Stabilization.
   - How is pricing determined?
     —How often are prices reviewed?
     —Why are prices increased or decreased?
     —Is your pricing competitive?
   - What have your price trends been like for the last three, five, and seven years?
   - How are your pricing policies viewed by:
     —Patients?
     —Referring physicians?
     —Insurers?
     —Competition?

5. **Accessibility:** Study your organization from the user's perspective; develop methods to improve accessibility to your products and services. If you have a quality product offered at the right price, good marketing dictates that you must offer that product in the right place. In most cases, patient convenience overrides all other concerns about products and services. However, accessibility is not just concerned with location. Other elements of accessibility include a reduced waiting time, a polite and respectful staff, and equipment that is designed to be nonthreatening. Creating an environment where patients want to be is as essential as making it easy for them to find you. See figure 3.5 for examples of accessibility strategies useful in meeting the convenience of your customers.

6. **Selling:** Personal selling, advertising, and public relations are the tasks necessary to inform existing and potential new cus-

Figure 3.5 Accessibility Strategies

Patient Need	Marketing Strategy
Parking	Free parking, valet parking, lighted lot
Public Transportation	Location on bus line
	Supply bus schedules.
Home Care	Arrange transportation.
	Offer a portable service.
Location	Operate satellite offices.
	Consider a mall outlet.
Convenient Time	Computerized scheduling system
	Extended hours

Adapted from Brown, S. W. and Morley, A. P. *Marketing Strategies for Physicians.* Oradell, NJ, Medical Economics Books. 1986, p.130.

Figure 3.6 Marketing Communication Elements

Source	Channel	Receiver
Radiologist	Newsletter	Present Patients
Manager	Educational Programs	Future Patients
Specialty	Paid Advertising	Referring Physicians
Association	Personal Contact	Employers
		Insurers

tomers about the available services. "Communication" is a more appropriate term to use when conveying the idea of "selling." The function of promotion is to let people know that you have a product or service to sell. Communicating that message involves three elements: a source, a channel, and a receiver. Figure 3.6 describes marketing communication elements and how they are interrelated.

7. **Evaluation:** A successful marketing plan requires that the services you provide be re-evaluated on a regular basis. Monitoring your program will involve determining satisfaction of referring physicians and patients. Program evaluation also entails the continuous monitoring of exam volumes, patient demographics, and referral patterns. Take the case of the "Disappearing Patients." A radiologist in a small community became worried about a decline in patient load. This decline seemed to correspond to the recent opening of a competing imaging center.

8. **Data:** Research and analysis of the service area yielded this representative marketing data:

- The average decline in exam volumes was 5 per week.
- Of surveyed patients, 60 percent complained about the office staff.
- Of surveyed patients, 50 percent stated that weekend and evening appointment times were desirable.
- Of female patients, 75 percent had received mammography at another center.
- Of those female patients, 60 percent stated they would have preferred to get their mammography at this radiologist's center.

9. **Goals:** The radiologist then developed specific marketing goals to address the issues uncovered by the market research.

   - Evaluate the customer relations skills of staff members and provide training in interpersonal skills.
   - Evaluate current office hours and make changes in those hours to improve accessibility.
   - Initiate a mammography program and acquire training in mammography interpretation.

10. **Strategies:** (See Figure 3.7)

    - Improve staff effectiveness.
      —Involve staff in planning for the center.
      —Conduct customer relations training.
      —Instill in each staff member a sense of responsibility for the overall success of the center.
    - Reconfigure hours of operation.
      —Begin extended hours two days per week.
      —Operate a Saturday morning schedule.
      —Arrange flexible staffing patterns to gain employee support and satisfaction with new hours.
    - Initiate a mammography service.
      —Acquire appropriate equipment and competent personnel.
      —Attend advanced training in mammographic techniques.

Training for Market Know-How

Most radiology managers will tell you that everything they know about marketing would fit into the space of a thimble. While the radiology manager may be bright, conscientious, and well-intend-

Figure 3.7 Top 10 Service Strategies for Boosting Referrals

- Extended office hours
- Special arrangements for patient transport
- Same-day or next-day service
- Fax and fax forms for patient scheduling
- Free mammography screenings
- Rapid report turnaround
- Educational mailers on imaging procedures (for patients)
- Educational newsletters on imaging technology (for physicians)
- Instructional presentations tailored to referral group
- Mobile services

Adapted from: Market-based strategies boost imaging referrals. *Diagnostic Imaging.* 15(1):23, 1993.

Figure 3.8 Factors that Influence Repeat Referral Business to MRI

- *Report turnaround:* Is the report done in a timely manner or has the patient phoned the referring physician before the report is available?
- *Guest relations:* Does the patient return to the referring physician with complaints of lack of dignity? Is the technology explained? Are the magnet's hammering noises explained? Can a family member sit in the scan room? Is the environment pleasant or is to too "high tech" and sterile-looking? Is the staff polite and helpful?
- *Location:* Is the center convenient for the patients? Is the site easy to find, are printed directions provided, or does the referring physician's office spend time giving directions?
- *Radiologist's reputation and film quality:* Is the center providing high-quality products?
- *Patient care issues:* Are the patients properly screened for ferrous objects? Are thorough histories taken?
- *Appointment scheduling:* Is there a wait for an appointment? Can the patient be scheduled outside of the 8 to 4 block on weekdays?
- *Patient transportation:* Is transportation available for the elderly or nonambulatory patient?
- *Educational programs:* Does the center radiologist keep the referring physicians apprised of innovations and new applications for MRI technology?
- *Specialization:* Is the center known for spine or pediatric work?
- *Pricing:* Is the pricing structure in line with the competition?*

*Hughes, C.M. MRI centers must sell themselves to survive in competitive market. *Diagnostic Imaging.* 10(7):95, 1988.

ing, he is probably a novice at healthcare marketing. The absence of marketing know-how in healthcare organizations is compensated for by the use of professional marketing firms specializing in hospital work. The combination of outside expert advice and inhouse planners and publicists is a situation that occurs frequently in healthcare. If you are a radiology manager in a general acute care hospital, you should notice that your administration is striving to become more market oriented.

As a manager you should increase your knowledge of services marketing in general, and study specific activities for medical imaging in detail. A fair knowledge of marketing can be acquired more quickly by attending seminars, workshops, and convention sessions offered by the professional organizations that serve the field of radiology. You can also enroll in regular or continuing education courses at your local college; you will find that marketing is a very popular major these days. Finally, network with your peers and seek out individuals who have a successful track record of marketing imaging services.

Overcoming the Negative Image of Marketing

Medical marketing has made great strides in the last decade. There is an increasing awareness within the healthcare industry that marketing, when professionally done, is an acceptable activity. Skeptical attitudes about marketing are a holdover from past beliefs that advertising in medicine was unprofessional and in poor taste. The skeptical attitudes stem from the implications that marketing is a foggy concept that's equated with the controversial components of advertising, promotion, and selling. Marketing in healthcare has become a fact of life—a necessary tool of survival in a very competitive business.

As stated earlier, marketing is viewed too narrowly. Physicians in particular often mistake a piece of marketing from the whole effort: "Marketing is just selling" or "Marketing is newspaper ads and billboards." The following discussion will help to dispel some myths about healthcare marketing. Dispelling these myths is based on the premise that marketing focuses an organization on the present and on the future services that it provides. The result of market planning is to offer services and products that the consuming public wants and needs. Let's look at these myths.

Marketing Is Just Advertising

Marketing is not just promotion and selling; marketing orients a provider to its consumers or constituencies. Effective marketing tells you who those consumers are, it prevents you from trying to sell surfboards in Antarctica, and it identifies the constituencies and their wants and needs. As a provider of imaging services there will be several constituencies; namely, the patient population, the referring physician, employers, government and social agencies, and insurers. Before the visible elements of promotion can begin, however, your house must be in order. Before the first ad appears, the following marketing processes must be set in motion:

- Know your customer.
- Set priorities for your services.
- Develop new services and enhance old services based on market research.
- Set appropriate fees.
- Locate your services conveniently.
- Agree on ethical promotional ideas.
- Promote an atmosphere of "hospitality."
- Concentrate on customer satisfaction and retention.

Marketing Is Just a Fancy Office

As healthcare professionals, our view of the services that we provide to our patients can be myopic; that is, too focused on the procedure. But the services we provide begin long before the radiologic examination. The service begins the moment that the patient picks up the phone and makes first contact with the office. This first impression will be the one that lasts, and this initial introduction to your services and products is often in the hands of a receptionist. The quality of that first interaction with the patient sets the tone for the visit. Take a look at some successful organizations with which you deal regularly; study the reception that you receive as a customer. Compare the behaviors you have observed as a customer to the practices used in greeting the public in your own workplace.

Visit the reception areas of your competitors. Note that the purpose of the space is "receiving," not "waiting." The reception area should be designed with patient needs in mind. Comfortable seating, good lighting, health education materials, and current magazines are some of the appointments that will make your reception area inviting. The comfortable and pleasant look of a reception area will influence the patient's perception about the quality and value of the services that he will receive.

Another major indicator of quality that patients use to judge the services that they have purchased is how the staff interacts with them. The quality of the time spent with the patient is enhanced with good eye contact, effective listening, and an empathetic caring attitude. These interpersonal interactions continue with billing personnel and follow-up phone calls to assess patient satisfaction.

Advertising Is Unprofessional

Tasteful marketing efforts are appropriate and educational for an increasingly more sophisticated healthcare consumer. Well-conceived promotional efforts are a public service that often teach the target audience to be better consumers by suggesting choices. Advertorial style print advertising is extremely useful for describing health risk factors for medical conditions such as cardiovascular disease or stroke. Public service announcements for breast self-examination will direct patients towards mammography screening programs. Free prostate screening will lead to an increase of referrals for ultrasound examinations. The increased competitiveness of healthcare today makes marketing a necessary evil of doing business. There is no need to feel guilty about marketing your services, but be sure to do it with good taste. Avoid quick promotions that simply copy trends in place at the time, be distinctive, and concentrate on developing a "share of mind" in your target audience that clearly delineates that your product is superior.

Marketing Is Someone Else's Responsibility

Marketing is everybody's business. One of the unique features of successful American companies, as reported in the best selling book *In Search of Excellence* by Tom Peters, is a "closeness to the customer," which is a customer-driven mentality that is held by each and every employee. The message is clear: all personnel must recognize that their jobs depend upon the success of the organization. Everyone has a personal stake in promoting customer satisfaction. Management's responsibility in this internal marketing initiative is to clearly communicate to all employees customer relations expectations. In behavioral terms, employees should be taught some simple rules of etiquette about responding to the needs of customers that will reap return business through goodwill.

- Be helpful to other employees; working together benefits the patient.
- Be cordial, smile and make eye contact.
- Respond quickly to requests for help.
- Protect the dignity of the patient.
- Be professional in appearance.
- Explain what you are doing.
- Listen attentively to complaints.
- Avoid excessive noise in the workplace.

Developing the Marketing Plan

There are five steps to the market planning process. These steps help you analyze and coordinate the services you offer, the way you provide the services, and the customers who receive them.

1. Identify your marketing goals.
2. Select your target audience.
3. Analyze what customers want and need.
4. Develop your marketing strategies.
5. Monitor your effectiveness.

Study the following example of a marketing plan to promote mammography services. Use this example plan to develop plans of your own.

Marketing Plan: Mammography Program

Marketing Goal
Improve women's healthcare services by providing greater access to mammography screening.

Marketing Research and Analysis
- 40,000 women die annually from breast cancer.
- The incidence of breast cancer is rising to 150,000 new cases per year.

- Women lack basic education about breast cancer.
- Women fear mammography; think that it hurts.
- There is a high cancellation rate for mammography appointments.
- Women do not routinely practice breast self-examination.

Target Audience
- Women with family history of breast cancer.
- Women over the age of 35.
- Spouses of women in high risk groups.

Product
Need: increased detection.
Strategy: mammography screening.

Need: education.
Strategy: patient education materials, out-reach education to women's groups.

Need: better compliance with accepted screening recommendations of the American Cancer Society.
Strategy: referring physician education, reminders of scheduled appointment times, and follow-up to assure re-examination at appropriate intervals.

Price
Need: an affordable pricing structure.
Strategy: evaluation of current procedures and determining what a screening exam should entail.

Need: financial counseling.
Strategy: Assist patients in filing insurance claims.

Need: a competitive pricing plan.
Strategy: Survey the market for comparative services and adjust pricing accordingly.

Place
Need: easy access to mammography services.
Strategy: conveniently located imaging center, extended hours, and weekend appointments.

Need: a comfortable environment.
Strategy: Create an interior design to women's tastes; use reading materials and educational brochures that cater to women's interests.

Promotion
Need: awareness of the risks of breast cancer.
Strategy: better communication with the public via lecture, television, radio, print advertising, or newsletters.
Strategy: Increase family involvement. Market directly to the spouses of women in high risk categories.

Benchmarks for Successful Marketing

As a provider you must focus on value and continuous improvement of the quality of the imaging services that you sell. In order to respond sensitively to your customers, concentrate on the following basic tenets:

1. Orientation towards total customer satisfaction.
2. Innovative practices that place the quality of your services ahead of the pack.
3. View your customers as partners.
4. Create value by fostering the perception of high quality through service excellence.

What You Can Do

Get involved in your community. Join civic organizations, volunteer, participate in public forums, and meet your community leaders.

Make the community aware of your services. Offer free services, provide professional services at public events, offer first aid at sporting events, do some public speaking, and contribute to local charities.

Become a member of your professional community. Join and participate in local professional societies, attend local social functions, become a member of the chamber of commerce.

Appear in print. Contribute articles to local school and church publications. Write a regular column in the local press; place your literature in your local "Welcome Wagon."

Finally, remember that everyone has a role to play. Each employee in an organization participates and contributes to overall marketing efforts. The success of your enterprise won't depend on just the radiologist, a piece of high technology, and a new building. Ultimately, what leads to success is superior service provided to patients by warm and caring people.

Appendix A

*Department of Radiology Physician Satisfaction Survey**

Hello! The purpose of this survey is to determine your satisfaction with the radiology department. Please take five minutes to fill out the questions below.

	SUPERIOR AGREE ALWAYS		POOR DISAGREE NEVER		
1. How frequently are you able to find a radiographic study?	1	2	3	4	5
2. How often do you hold films because you are concerned that a film will be lost once it is returned to radiology?	1	2	3	4	5
3. Are you satisfied with the radiology department in general?	1	2	3	4	5
4. Are you satisfied with the level of expertise of the radiologists?	1	2	3	4	5
5. Are you satisfied with the speed of dictated reports?	1	2	3	4	5
6. Are you satisfied with the level of technology available within the radiology department?	1	2	3	4	5
7. Do you ever delay reviewing studies secondary to the difficulty in finding films?	1	2	3	4	5

*Adapted from: Leckie, R. et. al. Surveying for Excellence in Radiology. *Administrative Radiology*, 12(8):34, 1992.

8. Please rate the helpfulness of:

the radiologist	1	2	3	4	5
the technologist	1	2	3	4	5
the file room clerk	1	2	3	4	5

9. Are you satisfied with the quality of the images produced?   1   2   3   4   5

10. How frequently are you able to retrieve films:
    <48 hours old?   1   2   3   4   5
    >48 hours old?   1   2   3   4   5

11. How available is the radiologist to review films with you?   1   2   3   4   5

12. What is the average amount of time spent finding a study?   <5'   10'   20'   >30'

13. How much time per day spent locating and evaluating films?   <10'   30'   1 hr   2 hr   >2 hr

14. What do you feel is the biggest source of complaint within the radiology department?

Appendix B

*Comparison of Questionnaires and Interviews**

Advantages of Questionnaires

- **Time saving to administer.** Self-administration reduces time; questionnaire can be designed to take limited time for busy physicians.
- **Standardization.** Written instructions reduce biases from differences in administration or from interactions with interviewer.
- **Anonymity.** Privacy encourages candid and honest responses to sensitive questions.

---

* Some material adapted with permission from Cummings SR, Strull W, Nevitt MC, Hulley SB. Planning the measurements: questionnaires. In: Hulley SB, Cummings SR, eds. *Designing Clinical Research: An Epidemiologic Approach.* Baltimore: Williams & Wilkins, 1988, p. 43. Used with the permission of Imaging Economics Newsletter. Vol. 1, No. 4, 1993, p.2.

- **Trending.** Written surveys with numerical scores facilitate comparison with repeat or follow-up surveys.

Disadvantages of Questionnaires
- **Time consuming to prepare.** Careful design and pretesting can be time consuming.
- **Can't correct for respondent error.** May be difficult to clarify response if respondent misunderstands or mismarks the questionnaire.

Advantages of Interviews
- **Clarity.** Interviewer can clarify questions.
- **Richness.** Interviewer can collect more complex answers and observations.
- **Completeness.** Interviewer can minimize missing and inappropriate responses.
- **Control.** Interviewer can control the order of questions.

Disadvantages of Interviews
- **Time consuming to administer.** Physician's and interviewer's time involved in administration.
- **Costly.** Includes interviewer's time.
- **May be incomplete.** May fail to elicit negative responses.
- **Nonconfidential.** Does not ensure anonymity desired by some physicians.

Appendix C

*Patient Satisfaction Survey**

1. Patient Information:

Age _____   Male _____
                                              Female ____

For what illness, injury, or condition were you sent to the radiology department? _____

Were you an inpatient (in the hospital)? _____

Were you an outpatient (not hospitalized)? _____

Were you an imaging center patient? _____

---

*Adapted from the American Healthcare Radiology Administrators, 1993.

2. Procedure performed:

On what part of the body was the procedure performed? _____

What type of procedure did you have?

____X-ray   ____MRI (Magnetic Resonance
                                          Imaging)

____Upper GI   ____Radiation Therapy

____Lower GI   ____Nuclear Medicine

____Computed Tomography   ____Cardiac Catheterization
       (CT scan, CAT scan)

____Ultrasound   ____Biopsy

____Other

Please circle, for the following, how satisfied you were with your
treatment in the Radiology Department.

		Least Satisfied			Most Satisfied
3. How satisfied were you with the concern, compassion, etc. shown to you by the following staff members?					
Receptionist	1	2	3	4	5
Technologist (who performed your test)	1	2	3	4	5
Radiologist (doctor) (if you saw one)	1	2	3	4	5

Comments: _____

_____

		Least Satisfied			Most Satisfied
4. How satisfied were you with the courteousness and friendliness shown to you by the following staff members?					
Receptionist	1	2	3	4	5

Technologist (who performed your test)	1	2	3	4	5
Radiologist (doctor) (if you saw one)	1	2	3	4	5

Comments: _____

_____

	Least Satisfied				Most Satisfied
5. How satisfied were you with the privacy given to you in the following?					
Changing area	1	2	3	4	5
Dressing gown	1	2	3	4	5
Discussion of your procedure	1	2	3	4	5
Privacy during your procedure	1	2	3	4	5

Comments: _____

_____

	Least Satisfied				Most Satisfied
6. How satisfied were you with the staff's attempt to meet your personal needs?					
Needing help to change into a gown	1	2	3	4	5
Needing physical assistance before or during procedure	1	2	3	4	5
Keeping family members informed	1	2	3	4	5
Special medical needs	1	2	3	4	5

Comments: _____

_____

		Least Satisfied				Most Satisfied
7.	How satisfied were you with the explanations given?					
	About forms to be filled out	1	2	3	4	5
	About what would happen during the procedure	1	2	3	4	5
	During procedure	1	2	3	4	5
	About what to expect after procedure	1	2	3	4	5

Comments: _____

_____

		Least Satisfied				Most Satisfied
8.	Please rate your overall satisfaction with your experience in our Radiology department including registration, reception, procedure, etc.	1	2	3	4	5

Comments: _____

_____

9. How long were you in the Radiology Department? _____

Were there any unusual delays? ____No   ____Yes

If there were any delays, were the delays explained? __Yes __No

Comments: _____

_____

10. What could we do better?

Comments: _____

_____

3.5 DIRECTORY OF RADIOLOGIC ORGANIZATIONS

This reference guide for radiologic organizations will be helpful to managers in need of specific information about the purposes of individual groups, continuing education opportunities, and sources of literature allied to the field of radiology. This listing was compiled from three different sources: *The 1992 Radiology Reference Guide*, Access Publishing Co.; *The 1992 Organization Directory*, Glendale Publishing Co.; and *Organizations in Radiology 1991*, American College of Radiology.

American Association of Healthcare Consultants (AAHC)
11208 Waples Mill Road, Suite 109, Fairfax, VA 22030
(703) 691-2242
Purpose: The American Association of Healthcare Consultants credentials members, helps clients select consultants, provides professional development, and enforces its Code of Ethics. When selecting consultants, it pays to consider the source.

American Association of Medical Dosimetrists (AAMD)
c/o Credentialling Services, Inc., P. O. Box 1498, Galesburg, IL 61401
(309) 343-1202
Purpose: The purposes of the Association are to promote the proper application of medical radiation dosimetry, to clarify and strengthen the position of dosimetrists within the radiation therapy community, to establish guidelines for the training and continuing education of dosimetrists, and to develop more direct lines of communication among dosimetrists.

American Association of Physicists in Medicine (AAPM)
335 East 45th Street, New York, NY 10017
(212) 661-9404
Purpose: The purposes of the American Association of Physicists in Medicine are to promote the application of physics to medicine and biology, to encourage interest and training in medical physics, and to prepare and desseminate technical information in this and related fields.

American Association for Women Radiologists (AAWR)
1891 Preston White Drive, Reston, VA 22091
(703) 648-8939
Purpose: The Association seeks to address socioeconomic issues unique to women in radiology, to serve as a resource organization for women in practice and as a support group for women in radiology residency, and to encourage participation of women at all levels in national radiological societies.

American Board of Nuclear Medicine
900 Veteran Ave., Los Angeles, CA 90024-1786
(310) 825-6787
Purpose: The primary purpose of the Board is the advancement of the health of the public through the establishment and maintenance of standards of training, education and qualifaction of physicians rendering care in nuclear medicine to the people of the United States.

The American Board of Radiology, Inc.
2301 West Big Beaver Road, Suite 625, Troy, MI 48084
(313) 643-0300
Purpose: The American Board of Radiology is a certifying organization for diagnostic radiologists and radiologic physicists.

American Cancer Society
1599 Clifton Road NE, Atlanta, GA 30329
(404) 382-7606
Purpose: This nationwide voluntary health organization is dedicated to eliminating cancer as a major health problem by preventing cancer, saving lives from cancer, and diminishing suffering from cancer through research, education, and service.

American College of Cardiology (ACC)
9111 Old Georgetown Rd., Bethesda, MD 20814
(301) 897-5400
Purpose: ACC is an international nonprofit professional medical society and teaching institution dedicated to cardiovascular care and disease prevention through professional education, promotion of research, and leadership in the development of standards of healthcare.

American College of Healthcare Executives (ACHE)
840 North Lake Shore Drive, Chicago, IL 60611
(312) 943-0544
Purpose: The American College of Healthcare Executives represents the leaders of the healthcare management profession and works toward the goal of bringing excellence to healthcare management.

American College of Medical Imaging
9465 Wilshire Blvd., #818, Beverly Hills, CA 90212
(213) 275-1393
Purpose: The American College of Medical Imaging is a medical association with an emphasis on continuing medical education for radiologists.

American College of Medical Physics
1891 Preston White Drive, Reston, VA 22091
(703) 648-8966
Purpose: The American College of Medical Physics was founded to enhance the quality of the practice of medical physics, to engage in professional activities for the benefit of the medical physics community, and to promote the continuing competence of practitioners of medical physics.

American College of Medicine
233 East Erie Street, Suite 710, Chicago, IL 60611
(312) 951-1400
Purpose: The American College of Medicine's goal is to provide physicians with new medical knowledge as it is emerging, and to update physicians on the procedures accepted as current in the practice of medicine and surgery.

American College of Nuclear Medicine
P. O. Box 175, Landisville, PA 17538
(717) 898-6006, Fax (717) 898-0713
Purpose: The purposes of the College are to advance the science of Nuclear Medicine, improve Nuclear Medicine service to the patient, study the socioeconomic aspects of the practice of Nuclear Medicine, and encourage improved and continuing education for practitioners of Nuclear Medicine and allied professional fields.

American College of Nuclear Physicians (ACNP)
1101 Connecticut Ave., Northwest, Suite 700,
Washington, DC 20036
(202) 857-1135
Purpose: The American College of Nuclear Physicians is an association of more than 1,500 physicians trained in the specialty of Nuclear Medicine. The organization was establised to advance the science of Nuclear Medicine through study, education, and improvement of the socioeconomic aspects of the practice.

American College of Physician Executives (ACPE)
4890 West Kennedy Blvd., Suite 200, Tampa, FL 33609
(800) 562-8088
Purpose: The purpose of the College is to provide educational programming and information services to physicians who have opted for management careers.

American College of Radiology (ACR)
1892 Preston White Drive, Reston, VA 22091
(703) 648-8900
Purpose: The American College of Radiology is the principal organization serving radiologists with programs that focus on the practice of radiology and the delivery of comprehensive radiological health services. These programs in medical sciences, education, and in practice management serve the public interest and the interests of the medical community in which radiologists serve in both diagnostic and therapeutic roles. The stated purposes of the ACR are to advance the science of radiology, to improve radiologic service to the patient, to study the economic aspects of the practice of radiology, and to encourage improved and continuing education for radiologists and allied fields.

American Healthcare Radiology Administrators (AHRA)
P. O. Box 334, Sudbury, MA 01779
(508) 443-7591
Purpose: The AHRA is a nonprofit educational association organized to promote the highest level of management practice in the administration of radiological sciences.

American Imaging Association (AIA)
1200 17th St., NW, Suite 400, Washington, DC 90036
(202) 296-9200
Purpose: The American Imaging Association is a trade association representing physician-owned diagnostic imaging facilities, mobile diagnostic services, associate physicians and other professionals dedicated to the conduct of high-quality, cost-effective imaging services throughout the country.

The AIA represents its members on the legislative front and on reimbursement issues facing the diagnostic imaging industry. It also provides a unique forum for the exchange of information and ideas regarding the imaging industry. Member programs and services include: Legislative Updates and Alerts, regional seminars, industry surveys, and group insurance programs.

American Institute of Ultrasound in Medicine (AIUM)
11200 Rockville Pike, Suite 205, Rockville, MD 20852-3139
(301) 881-2486, (800) 638-5352
Purpose: The American Institute of Ultrasound in Medicine (AIUM), founded in 1951, is dedicated to advancing the art and science of ultrasound in medicine and research. Its activities are professional, educational, literary, and scientific. AIUM's membership consists of more than 10,000 physicians, scientists, engineers, veterinarians, sonographers, technicians, manufacturers, manufacturers' representatives, and medical students.

American Institute of Physics
335 East 45th Street, New York, NY 10017
(212) 661-9404
Purpose: The American Institute of Physics is a not-for-profit membership corporation chartered in New York State in 1931 for the purpose of promoting the advancement and diffusion of the knowledge of physics and its application to human welfare.

American Medical Association (AMA)
515 North State St., 17th Floor, Chicago, IL 60610
(312) 464-5000
Purpose: The AMA is a voluntary service organization of physicians, more than 290,000 from every segment of medicine, whose mission is to promote the science and art of medicine and the betterment of public health.

American Osteopathic College of Radiology
119 East 2nd St., Milan, OH 63556
(816) 265-4011
Purpose: The purpose of the American Osteopathic College of Radiology is to: foster and maintain the highest possible standards in the specialty of radiology; further education of its members by the presentation of subjects of interest and courses of instruction and the publication of scientific data pertinent to radiology at such intervals as shall suit the needs of the membership; recognize the osteopathic concepts as they relate to the field of radiology; stimulate and maintain high morals and ethical standards in the specialty of radiology; and promote the public health.

American Radiological Nurses Association
2021 Spring Road, Suite 600, Oak Brook, IL 60521
(708) 571-9072
Purpose: The American Radiological Nurses Association exists to provide quality care in the diagnostic/therapeutic radiology environments.

American Radium Society (ARS)
1101 Market Street, 14th Floor, Philadelphia, PA 19107
(215) 574-3179
Purpose: The ARS is an organization of physicians and other scientists with common interest in cancer therapy. Its objectives are to promote the study of cancer in all its aspects, to encourage liaison among the various medical specialties concerned with the treatment of cancer, and to continue the scientific study of the treatment of the cancer patient.

American Registry of Clinical Radiology Technologists
710 Higgins Road, Park Ridge, IL 60064
(708) 318-9050
Purpose: The primary goal of this organization is to function as a national certifying agency for clinical radiologic technologists.

American Registry of Diagnostic Medical Sonographers (ARDMS)
2368 Victory Parkway, Suite 510, Cincinnati, OH 45206
(513) 281-7111, (800) 541-9754
Purpose: ARDMS is a nonprofit organization that administers voluntary certification examinations in diagnostic medical sonography and vascular technology.

The American Registry of Radiologic Technologists (ARRT)
1255 Northland Drive, Mendota Heights, MN 55120
(612) 687-0048
Purpose: The ARRT is the national certifying body for radiologic technologists.

American Roentgen Ray Society
1891 Preston White Drive, Reston, VA 22091
(703) 648-8992
Purpose: The objective of the American Roentgen Ray Society as stated in the constitution shall be the advancement of medicine through the science of radiology. In support of its objectives, the society holds an annual scientific meeting each spring. The official journal of the ARRS is the American Journal of Roentgenology, published monthly.

American Society of Clinic Radiologists
1514 Jefferson Hwy., New Orleans, LA 70121
(504) 838-3495
Purpose: The American Society of Clinic Radiologists is a nonprofit society composed of radiologist representatives of major multispecialty clinics with the common goal of maintaining and improving the quality and efficiency of radiologic care. Members meet with each other to share information about educational, operational, technical, political and socioeconomic aspects of radiologic practice, especially as related to large multispecialty groups.

American Society of Clinical Oncology
435 North Michigan Ave., Suite 1717, Chicago, IL 60611-4067
(312) 644-0828
Purpose: The American Society of Clinical Oncology is a society of clinical practitioners in the treatment of cancer.

American Society of Emergency Radiology (ASER)
1891 Preston White Drive, Reston, VA 22091
(703) 648-8982
Purpose: The purposes of the ASER are to advance and improve the radiologic aspects of emergent patient care; to establish emergency radiology as an area of special interest in the field of diagnostic imaging; to improve the methods of education in emergency radiol-

ogy; to provide a mechanism for presentation of scientific papers (through its meetings) on various aspects of emergency radiology; to promote research in emergency radiology; and to act as a resource body on emergency radiology for those interested in emergent patient care.

American Society of Head and Neck Radiology
2210 Midwest Road, Suite 207, Oak Brook, IL 60521
(708) 574-0660
Purpose: ASHNR was founded to stimulate interest and advance knowledge in the field of head and neck radiology, to improve methods of teaching radiologic diagnosis of disease of the head and neck, and to promote the dissemination of knowledge in head and neck radiology.

American Society of Neuroimaging
2221 University Ave., Suite 340, Minneapolis, MN 55414
(612) 378-7240, Fax (612) 623-3504
Purpose: The ASN is a professional, scientific organization comprised of all types of neuroscientists dedicated to the advancement of all types of neuroimaging. ASN's purposes include promotion and encouragement of the highest standards of neuroimaging.

American Society of Neuroradiology (ASN)
2210 Midwest Road, Suite 207, Oak Brook, IL 60521
(708) 574-0220
Purpose: The Society was established to develop and support standards for training in the practice of neuroradiology, to foster independent research, and to promote a close fellowship and exchange of ideas among neuroradiologists.

American Society of Radiologic Technologists (ASRT)
15000 Central Ave., Southeast, Albuquerque, NM 87123-3909
(505) 298-4500
Purpose: The American Society of Radiologic Technologists (ASRT) has been the preeminent national professional society for radiologic technologists for more than 70 years. As the national professional voice for radiologic technologists, the ASRT represents individual practitioners, educators, manager/administrators and students in radiography, radiation therapy, nuclear medicine, sonography, magnetic resonance, as well as the many specialties within each modality. There are nearly 18,000 members nationally and internationally.

The goals of the ASRT are to advance the professions of radiation and imaging specialties; to maintain high standards of education; to enhance the quality of patient care; and to further the welfare and socioeconomics of radiologic technologists.

Each year, the ASRT produces numerous regional specialty continuing education conferences and two large national programs. The Society also produces a variety of educational materials including self-study programs, videotapes, booklets, and audiotapes. It will pioneer in teleconferencing and lay the groundwork for educational offerings for technologists in AIDS awareness, geriatric special needs, the impact of OSHA in clinical settings and re-entry into the profession by inactive radiographers. As the national voice for radiologic technologists, the ASRT provides each member with the opportunity to chart the future of their profession.

American Society for Therapeutic Radiology & Oncology (ASTRO)
1891 Preston White Drive, Reston, VA 22091
(703) 648-8900
Purpose: The purposes of the Society are to extend the benefits of radiation therapy to patients with cancer or other disorders; to advance its scientific basis; and to provide for the education and professional fellowship of its members.

American Thoracic Society
1740 Broadway, New York, NY 10019-4374
(212) 315-8700
Purpose: Professional society of physicians and scientists involved in all aspects of pulmonary medicine and drug-related research.

American Urological Association, Inc.
1120 North Charles Street, Baltimore, MD 21201
(301) 727-1100
Purpose: The American Urological Association, Inc. specializes in sponsoring continuing medical education for urological physicians.

Association for Independent Medical Service
P. O. Box 55631, Houston, TX 77255
(800) 292-AIMS
Purpose: The Association for Independent Medical Service is a nonprofit organization consisting of executives and professionals in companies who install major medical equipment.

Association for the Advancement of Medical Instrumentation
Suite 400, 3330 Washington Blvd., Washington, DC 22201-0793
(703) 525-4890
Purpose: AAMI is a unique alliance of individuals from the healthcare professions who are united by the common goal of increasing the understanding and beneficial use of medical devices and instrumentation.

Association of American Medical Colleges
One DuPont Circle, N.W., Washington, DC 20036
(202) 828-0400
Purpose: The AAMC is an organization whose membership is comprised of accredited medical schools throughout the country. The association works with its members to set a national agenda for medical education, biomedical research, and health care.

Association of Educators in Radiological Sciences (AERS)
730 North LaSalle, Suite 1061, Chicago, IL 60610
(501) 972-3073
Purpose: The purposes of the Association are: 1) to advance the science of radiologic technology; 2) to assist in establishing and maintaning high standards of education and training; 3) to encourage the exchange of educational concepts and methodologies at all program levels of radiologic technology and related specialty areas; 4) to stimulate interest in academic advancement and teaching as a career option; 5) to advance the profession of radiologic technology and its related areas through encouragement of its members to conduct research and disseminate their works through publication; and 6) to foster mutual cooperation and understanding between radiologic technology educators and other external groups.

Association of Freestanding Radiation Oncology Centers
3960 Park Blvd., Suite E, San Diego, CA 92103
(619) 692-1598
Purpose: National network of physicians, physicists, managers and clinical personnel working in freestanding radiation oncology centers.

Association of Residents in Radiation Oncology
1101 Market St, 14th Floor, Philadelphia, PA 19107
(215) 574-3155
Purpose: The objectives of the Association of Residents in Radiation Oncology are to formalize resident input into professional organiza-

tions affecting radiation oncology residents, and to disseminate information to and foster communication among, residents.

Association of University Radiologists (AUR)
Johns Hopkins School of Public Health and Hygiene, 615 North Wolfe St., Baltimore, MD 20295
(301) 955-3350
Purpose: The Association was organized to promote full-time academic radiology. Its purposes are to encourage excellence in laboratory and clinical investigation, teaching and clinical practice; to stimulate interest in academic radiology as a career; to advance radiology as a medical science and to provide a forum in which university-based radiologists can present and discuss the results of research, teaching and administrative problems.

British Institute of Radiology
36 Portland Place, London, England, W1N 4AT
(071) 580-4085
Purpose: The British Institute of Radiology is a multidisciplinary learned society devoted to the radiological sciences.

Canadian Association of Medical Radiation Technologists
294 Albert St., Suite 601, Ottawa, Ontario, Canada K1P 6E6
(613) 234-0012
Purpose: The Canadian Association of Medical Radiation Technologists functions as the qualifying body for technologists in diagnostic and therapeutic radiology, as well as nuclear medicine, in Canada.

Canadian Association of Physicists Medical and Biological Physics Division
151 Slater St., Suite 903, Ottawa, Ontario, Canada K1P 5H3
(613) 237-3392
Purpose: The division's primary concerns are to promote and encourage the application of physics to medical and biological problems and to advance the scientific and professional interest of the members.

Canadian Association of Radiologists
1440 St. Catherine St., W., Suite 506, Montreal, Quebec, Canada H3G 1R8
(514) 866-2035
Purpose: The Canadian Association of Radiologists is charged with both the scientific advancement of the specialty, as well as its

socioeconomic concerns. Its objectives are to advance the art and science of radiology and to promote its interest in relation to medicine, with particular reference to the clinical, educational, ethical, and economic aspects thereof.

Center for the Advancement of Radiation Education and Research (CARER)
Johns Hopkins School of Public Health and Hygiene, 615 North Wolfe St., Baltimore, MD 21205
(301) 955-3350
Purpose: The Center for the Advancement of Radiation Education and Research (CARER) provides expert, credible, and objective information about the benefits and risks of radiation. CARER conducts educational programs and serves as a resource center for information concerning the use of radiation in medicine, industry, and energy production.

Committee on Allied Health Education and Accreditation
515 North State Street, 7th Floor, Chicago, IL 60610
(312) 464-4660
Purpose: The Committee on Allied Health Education and Accreditation (CAHEA) is a programmatic postsecondary accrediting agency recognized by the U. S. Secretary of Education and the Council on Postsecondary Accreditation and carries out its accrediting activities in cooperation with 20 review committees. CAHEA is sponsored by the American Medical Association and is the final deliberative body for the assessment of compliance with established standards for accreditation of educational programs for the allied health professions involved.

Complete Mammographic Technology
105 Pennicott Drive, Penfield, NY 14526
(716) 442-8432
Purpose: Responding to the educational needs of radiologic technologists doing mammography, this group was formed to provide practical solutions to meet the increased responsibility that is now given to the mammographer.

Computerized Medical Imaging Society
Georgetown University Medical Center, 3900 Reservoir Rd., NW, Washington, DC 20007
(202) 687-2121

Purpose: The Computerized Medical Imaging Society serves as a source for the exchange of information concerning the medical use of computerized tomography in radiological diagnosis.

Conference of Radiation Control Program Directors
71 Fountain Place, Frankfort, KY 40601
(502) 227-4543
Purpose: The purpose of the Conference is to function as a federal-state liaison for radiation control programs in the United States.

Council of Affiliated Regional Radiation Oncology Societies
1891 Preston White Drive, Reston, VA 22091
(703) 648-8938
Purpose: The council, through its network of 30 constituent organizations, provides a mechanism for the exchange and dissemination of information pertaining to the clinical practice of radiation oncology on a national level. The council also provides an alternate pathway to membership and fellowship in the American College of Radiology (ACR).

Eastern Radiological Society
Department of Radiology, Greenville Memorial Hospital, 701 Grove Rd., Greenville, SC 29605
(803) 242-7107
Purpose: The objective of the Eastern Radiological Society is to establish an organization of physicians-radiologists for the purpose of improving radiologic service by means of joint conferences and discussion groups.

Fleischner Society
5665 Oberlin Drive, Suite 110, San Diego, CA 92121
(619) 453-6222
Purpose: The Fleischner Society emphasizes a multidisciplinary approach to the diagnosis of chest disease. In addition to pulmonary radiologists, society members include experts in respiratory anatomy, pathology, physiology, clinical pulmonology, pediatrics, anesthesia and thoracic surgery. Many course sessions are designed to discuss chest disease from several points of view, often including anatomy, pathology, physiology, radiology, and clinical management.

Florida Radiological Society
3134-100 Lonnbladh Road, Tallahassee, FL 32308
(904) 422-1664, (800) 338-5901, Fax (904) 422-0047

Purpose: The Florida Radiological Society is a state chapter of the American College of Radiology. Its purpose is to further education through communication with radiological professionals.

Friends of the National Library of Medicine
1529 Wisconsin Ave., Washington, DC 20007
(202) 342-5563
Purpose: The Friends of the National Library are dedicated to increasing awareness and support for the library. This nonprofit organization promotes and publicizes the National Library of Medicine, the largest source of medical information in the world.

Health Physics Society
8000 Westpark Dr., Suite 400, McLean, VA 22102
(703) 790-1745
Purpose: The Health Physics Society's primary objective is the development of scientific knowledge and practical means for the protection of man and his environment from the harmful effects of radiation.

Independent X-Ray Dealers Association
111 East Wacker Dr., Suite 600, Chicago, IL 60601
(312) 644-6610
Purpose: An association of independent x-ray dealers who work to consistently improve, by education, exchange of information, ideas and joint cooperation, the professional field of radiology. Dedicated to the advancement of x-ray dealers in the United States.

Institute for Clinical PET
2105 National Press Building, Washington, DC 20045
(202) 466-4274
Purpose: Formed by nuclear medicine physicians, cardiologists, neurologists and radiologists, the Institute is the only nonprofit organization comprised of the leading multidisciplinary medical imaging physicians, scientists, administrators, and technologists representing PET centers and facilities around the world.

Institute of Applied Physiology & Medicine
701 16th Ave., Seattle, WA 98122
(206) 442-7330, Fax (206) 422-1717
Purpose: The Institute is a private, nonprofit organization dedicated to bringing new research developments into medical practice in such areas as cardiovascular and cerebrovascular physiology and cancer treatment therapy.

Interamerican College of Radiology
P.O. Box 650843, Miami, FL 33165
(305) 674-9838
Purpose: The Interamerican College of Radiology is an organization of radiologists in all countries of the Americas. The purpose of the college is to foster relationships and share in advances of radiology among radiologists of North, Central, and South America and throughout the rest of the world as well.

International Intradiscal Therapy Society (IITS)
P.O. Box 679, Grayslake, IL 60030-0679
(708) 223-2684, (800) 426-4868
Purpose: IITS is a nonprofit, ACCCME accredited, medical educational society dedicated to the research and treatment of intervertebral disc disorders.

International Organization for Medical Physics
Gershenson Radiation Oncology Center, Harper Hospital
3990 John R. Street, Detroit, MI 48201
(313) 745-2489
Purpose: The objectives of the International Organization for Medical Physics are to organize international cooperation in medical physics and to promote communication among the various branches of medical physics and allied subjects, to contribute to the advancement of medical physics in all its aspects, and to encourage and advise on the formation of national organizations of medical physics in those countries that lack such organizations.

International Skeletal Society
3400 Spruce St., Philadelphia, PA 19104
(215) 662-3019
Purpose: The International Skeletal Society is a nonprofit society of skeletal radiologists and individuals in related fields of medicine and science. The group advances the science and art of skeletal radiology through meetings, papers and courses.

The International Society for Optical Engineering (SPIE)
P.O. Box 10, Bellingham, WA 98227-0010
(206) 676-3290
Purpose: SPIE is a nonprofit society dedicated to advancing engineering and scientific applications of optical, electro-optical and optoelectronic instrumentation, systems, and technology. Its mem-

bers are scientists, engineers, and users interested in the reduction to practice of these technologies. SPIE provides the means for communicating new developments and applications to the scientific, engineering, and user communities through its publications and symposia.

International Society of Radiographers and Radiological Technicians
52 Addison Crescent, Don Mills, Ontario, Canada M3B1K8
(416) 445-7841
Purpose: The chief purpose of the International Society of Radiographers and Radiological Technicians is to promote and encourage improved standards of training in radiography, radiotherapy and allied subjects.

International Society of Radiology
c/o Professor W. A. Fuchs, Department of Radiology, University Hospital, CH-8091, Zurich, Switzerland
Purpose: The International Society of Radiology is the world organization of radiologists. Its members are the national radiological bodies, rather than individual radiologists. Radiological associations in 63 countries seek to help coordinate the progress of medical radiology, to undertake business referred to the ISR by member societies, and to provide financial support for the work of its commissions. The necessary financial resources are obtained by membership fees of the various national societies as well as by contributions from the International Congress of Radiology.

Joint Review Committee on Education in Diagnostic Medical Sonography (JRC DMS)
20 North Wacker Drive, Suite 900, Chicago, IL 60606
(312) 704-5151
Purpose: JRC DMS, in cooperation with the Committee on Allied Health Education and Accreditation, is responsible for educational programs in diagnostic medical sonography.

Los Angeles Radiological Society
P.O. Box 91215, Los Angeles, CA 90009-1215
(213) 642-0921
Purpose: The Los Angeles Radiological Society is an organization of diagnostic radiologists and radiation oncologist technologists. The society offers quality educational meetings for professionals.

Magnetic Resonance Managers Society (MRMS)
5856 Leesburg Pike, Bailey's Crossroads, VA 22041
(703) 931-1177
Purpose: MRMS is the only professional organization dedicated exclusively to serving managers of MRI facilities. The main thrust of the organization is to provide education and networking for its members.

Medical Records Institute
P.O. Box 289, Newtonville, MA 02160
(617) 964-3923
Purpose: The Medical Records Institute is an educational publishing company that conducts seminars, conferences, and workshops on improving records management.

Mid-Atlantic Society of Radiation Oncologists
Ridge Station, P.O. Box 29237, Richmond, VA 23229
(804) 786-0490
Purpose: MASRO was founded to provide a forum for the interaction of its members, a forum for scientific and educational interaction, and a forum to evaluate the socioeconomic forces operating on the specialty of radiation oncology.

Nancy Gosselin Foundation
8200 East Bellview, #700, Englewood, CO 80111
(303) 972-1706
Purpose: The purpose of the foundation is to provide educational and supportive services to the community about breast and other women's health issues. This includes offering education programs to healthcare professionals addressing women's health care issues.

National Computer Graphics Association
2722 Merrilee Dr., Suite 200, Fairfax, VA 22031
(703) 698-9600
Purpose: The National Computer Graphics Association is an organization of individuals and major companies dedicated to developing and promoting the computer graphics industry and to improving applications in business, government, science, and the arts.

National Consortium of Breast Centers (NCBC)
c/o Patty Wilcox, R.N., C. ANP, The Johns Hopkins Oncology Center, 550 North Broadway, Suite 1003, Baltimore, MD 21205
(301) 955-4850

Purpose: The goal of the National Consortium of Breast Centers is to foster excellence in the provision of breast healthcare services through multidisciplinary networking and educational seminars at annual meetings as well as through information shared through the NCBC newsletter, "The Breast Center Bulletin." The Consortium is focused primarily on helping professionals working in the breast healthcare arena as well as on connecting with the breast healthcare services available nationwide.

National Council on Radiation Protection and Measurement
7910 Woodmont Avenue, Suite 800, Bethesda, MD 20814
(301) 657-2652
Purpose: The NCRP provides the means by which nationally recognized scientific experts can bring their extensive ability, experience, and judgement to bear on all of the problems of radiation protection and measurement.

National Medical Association, Inc.
c/o Elizabeth Patterson, M.D., Department of Radiology, University Hospital of Pennsylvania, 3400 Spruce St., Philadelphia, PA 19104
(215) 662-4000
Purpose: The purposes of the National Medical Association, Section on Radiology are to provide a scientific forum, with an emphasis on the role of the minority radiologist, with an interest in education and training, socioeconomic problems and recognition of achievement, and to represent black radiologists' views in national activities.

New England Roentgen Ray Society
Massachusetts General Hospital, Boston, MA 02114
(617) 726-8763
Purpose: New England Roentgen Ray Society is a regional educational and scientific radiology society founded in 1915 that sponsors monthly scientific meetings and annual refresher courses on timely topics in imaging.

North American Hyperthermia Group
1891 Preston White Drive, Reston, VA 22091
(703) 648-3780
Purpose: The purpose of the North American Hyperthermia Group is to facilitate interaction and communication between theoreticians, experimentalists, and clinical practitioners from the disciplines of

physical and engineering sciences, biological and chemical sciences, and clinical and medical sciences that contribute to the understanding and use of hyperthermia; to promote basic research and the clinical application of hyperthermia; and to promote the diffusion of knowledge of hyperthermia to persons in the diverse disciplines interested in the fields of hyperthermia.

North American Society for Cardiac Imaging
c/o Lawrence Boxt, M.D., Secretary-Treasurer, Department of Radiology, Columbia Presbyterian Medical Center, 177 Fort Washington Avenue, New York, NY 10032
(212) 305-8264
Purpose: The Society was created to further the advancement of cardiac imaging. The Society is interdisciplinary, including radiologists, cardiologists and physicists.

North American Society of Cardiac Radiology
Department of Radiology, Little Company of Mary Hospital, 4101 Torrance Blvd, Torrance, CA 90503
(213) 540-7676 ext. 4840
Purpose: The North American Society for Cardiac Radiology was founded for the scientific advancement of cardiac imaging. Although the society is composed primarily of cardiac radiologists, there is strong representation from the fields of cardiology, nuclear medicine, ultrasound, cardiac pathology, physiology, and physics.

Radiation Research Society
1892 Preston White Drive, Reston VA 22091
(703) 648-3780
Purpose: The Society's purposes are to promote original research in the natural sciences relating to radiation, to facilitate integration of different disciplines in the study of radiation effects, and to promote the diffusion of knowledge in these fields.

Radiological Society of North America (RSNA)
2021 Spring Road, Suite 600, Oak Brook, IL 60521
(708) 571-2670
Purpose: The Radiological Society of North America is the largest association of radiologists and physicists in medicine, dedicated exclusively to scientific education and the provision of continuing education opportunities in the radiological health sciences.

Radiology Business Management Association (RBMA)
27241 LaPaz Road, Suite 120, Laguna Niguel, CA 92656
(714) 833-1651
Purpose: The cornerstones of RBMA can be summed up in four basic objectives: 1) recognition and enhancement of the professionalism of radiology practice management; 2) improvement and expansion of services to radiologists and their managers in response to changing needs and requirements; 3) availability of information to members in ways to produce efficient communications; 4) quality educational programs designed to improve administrative skills.

Radiology Outreach Foundation
3415 Sacramento Street, San Francisco, CA 94118
(415) 564-3966
Purpose: The purpose of the Radiology Outreach Foundation is to provide radiological equipment, books, consultation, training, and education to healthcare practitioners in medically disadvantaged countries.

Radiology Research and Education Foundation
3415 Sacramento Street, San Francisco CA 94118
(415) 564-3966
Purpose: The purpose of the Radiology Research and Education Foundation is to support research and educational endeavors in radiology. It attracts donations from philanthropists, from industry, from alumni, and from academic staff. A separate Research Evaluation Committee does a review of all requests for funding and decides the allocation of resources the Board allots for the fiscal year. The committee uses an NIH scoring system; proposed investigations must pass rigorous scientific tests of credibility and value to receive funding. Grants and fellowships funded by the RREF last year totalled $1.5 million, and the total funded since it began in 1974 until last year was $5.5 million.

Royal Australasian College of Radiologists
37 Lower Fort St., Milers Point NSW 2000
Purpose: The purpose of the Royal Australasian College of Radiologists is to promote, encourage, and provide for the advancement of the study and the practice of the sciences known as diagnostic radiology and diagnostic medical imaging, therapeutic radiology

and oncology and allied sciences and for carrying out of research and experimental work in connection with these sciences.

Royal College of Radiologists
38 Portland Place, London W1N 3DG
Purpose: The purpose of the Royal College of Radiologists is to advance the science and practice of radiology and to establish and maintain the highest standards of practice. It is also the aim of the college to promote and publish research in radiology and related subjects. The college is responsible for approving all postgraduate training programs in radiology in the United Kingdom, conducting an examination, the Fellowship of the Royal College of Radiologists, and accrediting radiologists who have completed their postgraduate training. The college embraces radiodiagnosis, as well as radiotherapy and oncology, and their allied sciences.

Society for Cardiac Angiography & Interventions
P.O. Box 7849, Breckenridge, CO 80424
(303) 453-1773
Purpose: Dedicated to fostering excellence in cardiac imaging, the Society encourages clinical diagnostic research, defines and maintains quality and training standards, and promotes constructive interaction and peer assessment among practitioners.

Society for Magnetic Resonance Imaging (SMRI)
213 West Institute Place, Suite 501, Chicago, IL 60610
(312) 751-2590
Purpose: The SMRI purposes are: to provide an opportunity to physicians and basic scientists to contribute to the development of MRI as a diagnostic technique in medicine and biology, with special emphasis on imaging; and to provide an international, multi-disciplinary forum for the advancement of MRI.

Society for Pediatric Radiology
600 Grant Street, 6th Fl., Denver, CO 80203-3527
(303) 831-6579, Fax (303) 866-9488
Purpose: Purposes of the Society include the study of problems associated with the practice of pediatric radiology, the education of members and others in regard to these problems, and the association of persons professionally concerned with such problems.

Society for Radiation Oncology Administrators (SROA)
2021 Spring Road, Suite 600, Oak Brook, IL 60521
(708) 571-9065
Purpose: The Society is a national organization whose objectives are to improve the administration of the business and nonmedial management aspects of radiation oncology, and the practice of radiation oncology as a cost effective form of healthcare delivery, to provide a forum for dialogue between the members on matters of professional interest, to disseminate information among members of the society, and to generally promote the field of radiation oncology administration.

The Society for Radiologists in Ultrasound
1101 Market Street, 14th Floor, Philadelphia, PA 19107
(215) 274-3183
Purpose: The Society was established for the purpose of the advancement of ultrasound. The society has an international membership and is a specific, professional, and educational organization.

Society of Breast Imaging
33 Old Connecticut Path, Wayland, MA 01778
(617) 956-0045
Purpose: The Society of Breast Imaging is a society of radiologists with clinical and/or academic recognition in the area of breast imaging.

Society of Cardiovascular and Interventional Radiology (SCVIR)
10201 Lee Highway, Suite 160, Fairfax, VA 22030
(703) 691-1805
Purpose: SCVIR is a nonprofit, national scientific organization committed to its mission to improve health and the quality of life through the practice of cardiovascular and interventional radiology. The Society promotes education, research, and communication in the field while providing strong leadership in the development of healthcare policy.

Society of Chairmen of Academic Radiology Departments (SCARD)
c/o David Levin, M. D., Secretary-Treasurer, Department of Radiology, Thomas Jefferson University Hospital, 130 South 9th Street, Suite 1004 Edison, Philadelphia, PA 19107
(215) 955-7264

Purpose: The purposes of SCARD are to promote medical education, research, and patient care, particularly as concerns radiology; develop teaching methods of graduate and undergraduate radiology; and to provide a forum for discussion of problems and developments of mutual interest and free informal interchange of ideas among departmental chairmen of academic radiology departments.

Society of Chairmen of Academic Radiation Oncology Programs
1101 Market St., 14th Floor, Philadelphia, PA 19107
(215) 574-3164

Purpose: The special objectives of the Society of Chairmen of Academic Radiation Oncology Programs are directed toward the advancement of the art and science of radiation oncology. This is done by promoting medical education, research, and patient care in radiation oncology in addition to developing methods and teaching radiotherapy to undergraduates and graduates. The society provides a means for discussing problems and developments of mutual interest and concern with free and informal exchange of ideas among the program chairmen of radiation oncology.

Society of Computed Body Tomography
P.O. Box 1026, Rochester, MN 55903-1026
(206) 543-3320

Purpose: The Society was founded for the purpose of the scientific, educational, and professional advancement of computed body tomography.

Society of Diagnostic Medical Sonographers (SDMS)
12225 Greenville Ave., Suite 434, Dallas, TX 75243
(214) 235-7367

Purpose: SDMS is the professional society for diagnostic ultrasonographers. Its primary purpose is to promote education in diagnostic medical sonography.

Society of Gastrointestinal Radiologists
University of Washington, Seattle, WA 98185
(206) 543-0871

Purpose: The Society promotes the educational process in radiology and gastrointestinal radiology through accredited continuing medical education programs.

Society of Magnetic Resonance in Medicine (SMRM)
1918 University Ave., Suite 3C, Berkeley, CA 94704
(510) 841-1899
Purpose: The Society of Magnetic Resonance in Medicine is an international, nonprofit professional association devoted to the promotion of research and education in all applications of magnetic resonance in medicine and biology. The SMRM is, at present, the only medical society that combines these multiple disciplines in order to best serve medicine and science.

Society of Nuclear Medicine, Inc. (SNM)
136 Madison Avenue, New York, NY 10016
(212) 889-0717
Purpose: The Society of Nuclear Medicine is incorporated as a nonprofit corporation for scientific, education, and philanthropic purposes. The objectives of the Society are 1) to establish and maintain an organization of physicians and scientists of high standing with a common interest in the scientific and clinical disciplines concerned with the diagnostic, therapeutic, and investigational use of radionuclides; 2) to foster meetings of the organization for the purpose of communicating and discussing knowledge of nuclear phenomena as they apply to the better understanding and control of disease; 3) to disseminate information concerning nuclear medicine by sponsoring scientific and professional publications; 4) to strive to better the welfare of mankind by maintaining and advancing the highest possible standards of education, research and practice of nuclear medicine; and 5) to address in a timely manner socioeconomic issues and government relations that may significantly affect the quality of education, research, and clinical practice in nuclear medicine.

Society of Thoracic Radiology
c/o Sanford A. Rubin, M. D., Department of Radiology, G-09, University of Texas Medical Branch, Galveston, TX 77550
(409) 772-3649
Purpose: The purposes of the Society are to foster thoracic radiology as an organized subspecialty in radiology; to represent thoracic radiology's interest at national and international levels; to develop and support standards for the teaching and practice of thoracic

radiology; to provide an open forum for thoracic radiologists to exchange ideas, stimulate research, disseminate knowledge and to develop and promote relationships with nonradiologic thoracic specialties.

Society of Uroradiology
c/o Jeffrey Newhouse, M.D., Room 2-125, 177 Ft. Washington Ave., New York, NY 10032
(212) 305-7898
Purpose: The Society of Uroradiology was established for the advancement of urinary tract imaging.

Society of Vascular Technology
1101 Connecticut Ave. NW, Suite 700, Washington, DC 20036-4303
(202) 847-1149
Purpose: The purpose of the Society is to support and promote the profession of vascular technology through programs and services in the areas of education, intersocietal relations, leadership and government relations.

Southern Association for Oncology
P.O. Box 190088, Birmingham, AL 35219-0088
(205) 942-0530
Purpose: The Southern Association for Oncology was established in 1987 to enhance the communication and interaction of practicing oncologists in all disciplines, with the ultimate goals of fostering practical medical education and improving the quality of oncological research, diagnosis, care, and understanding.

3.6 POLICIES AND PROCEDURES

General Principles

Every organization, from the local plastic wares dealer to the largest corporation, has policies and procedures to govern its activities. Often, they concern simple operating rules, unwritten codes of conduct, or routine matters. "The way we've always done it" is an axiom that can no longer be accepted in today's radiology department.

Policies and procedures provide the basis for efficient management practices by establishing important guides to assist the manager in decision making. If management can be described as a series of decision-making situations, then the judgements managers make must largely depend on carefully written statements of policy. To be effective, policies and procedures must be formally written to ensure uniformity and compliance. Standards of operation are clearly stated in terms that can be understood and interpreted. See figure 3.9 for the administrative procedures of policy management.

Figure 3.9 Policy Management

		MANAGEMENT POLICY
COMPANY/LOCATION		**STANDARD PROCEDURE**

SUBJECT	DERARTMENT	NUMBER
		PAGE
Policy Management	Radiology	
TITLE	DATE EFFECTIVE	DATE REVISED
Preparation of Policies and Procedures	APPROVED BY (Signature)	APPROVED BY (Signature)

```
                              POLICY
          PURPOSE:    The Radiology Department manager is respon-
                      sible for developing and maintaining policies
                      and procedures that document its operation.
                      There are three purposes for establishing
                      this framework:
                      A.  To provide detailed documentation of
                          department operations.
                      B.  To have available "how to" information for
                          employee training and reference.
                      C.  To communicate desired methods of interde-
                          partment operation and coordination.
          A manual should be maintained by the department director. This
          manual should include policies and procedures written for the
          Radiology Department and   those distributed by other
          departments which affect radiology. The manual should be
```

Figure 3.9 Policy Management (cont.)

---

separated into appropriate sections with tab dividers. The radiology manager is responsible for adding, revising, and correcting those policies and procedures.

PROCEDURE

PURPOSE: To provide guidelines for writing effective policies and procedures.

STANDARD FORM: Each policy and/or procedure should have a standard cover sheet. If a policy requires more than one typewritten page, or the policy is followed by any operating procedures, plain second sheets may be used.

PREPARATION OF
POLICIES AND
PROCEDURES: A <u>policy</u> is a set of guidelines establishing the boundaries within which action is to be taken. A <u>procedure</u> is a statement of who, what, when, where, how, and in what order action is taken. When writing policies and procedures, the following steps are taken:

1. Complete the heading information.
   a. Classify the policy and/or procedure by the subject addressed.
   b. Title the document according to its specific topic.
   c. Record the name of the department or section responsible for maintaining the document.
   d. Number the document in accordance with an established system.
   e. Enter the date that the original version of the document was or will be published.
   f. If the document is new, enter "None" in the "Date Revised" block. Otherwise, enter the effective date of the revision.
2. A policy should contain a purpose and any points needed to clarify or define constraints.
3. A procedure should always contain a purpose plus the detailed steps required to complete the tasks involved. In addition, the following information may optionally be included:
   a. <u>Frequency</u>. If the procedure should be performed at a certain time each day, week, or year, then this should be stated. The procedure could also be performed in case some other event, problem, or emergency occurs.

Figure 3.9   Policy Management (cont.)

---

   b. <u>Authority</u>. If the procedure must be performed by an
employee having a specific job title, this should be
included. If an employee must get permission to perform
the task or must notify the supervisor before or after
the task, then this should be stated.

   c. <u>Materials Required</u>. Documentation should be included
if an employee is required to use certain materials,
supplies, and equipment in order to meet standard
practice.

   d. <u>Precautions</u>. If there are hazards involved in the job,
then these should be specifically pointed out. Also,
common errors that have been observed to occur can be
identified so that they can be avoided in the future.
Any exceptions to normal performance of the procedure
should be noted. It would be useful to include a note
on anything that could harm the patient, the employee,
the building, or a piece of equipment.

   e. <u>Quality Expectations</u>. If there is some degree of
neatness, cleanliness, completeness, or accuracy that
is required and can be measured or observed, then it
can be noted.

   f. <u>Standard Time</u>. If there is an average time in which the
department director or supervisor believes that the
task could be completed, then this can be included.

Establishing Policies

Policies are guidelines for managerial action. Like plans, they are
both specific and general, short-term and long-term, and help accomplish the objectives of the organization. Policy-making is a
planning function. Policy statements ensure that action is oriented
towards objectives. Imagine taking a road trip without a map; when
trying to manage without the structure of policy, the behavior of
persons in your environment is strained and without direction. Like
the road trip without the map, consider how many deviations off
course can occur before a task is accomplished.

Policies and procedures are developed to achieve consistency and
direction and to protect the organization. In industry, the goals of
policies are consistent output and quality of product. In healthcare,

the goal is no different. Our view of the product, however, is a more complex matter. Effective policy-making requires recognition that there are many facets to successful policy management. Some essential criteria for effective policy-making are the following:

1. **Flexibility**   A policy needs to strike a delicate balance between being specific yet flexible enough to accommodate changes in conditions. The judgement of management determines this balance on a case-by-case basis.
2. **Comprehensiveness**   A policy should be comprehensive enough to cover any contingency. The comprehensiveness depends on the scope of actions that will be controlled. A policy may control a narrow range of activities such as hiring or be detailed enough to guide functions like public relations.
3. **Coordination**   Often a policy will coordinate the actions of various interrelated units. Without the coordinative direction that the policy provides, coming together for a common aim would be much more difficult. Policies dictating action for entities involved in disaster preparedness or fire safety are good examples of this coordinating function.
4. **Ethics**   A policy needs to conform to society's ethical standards. Managers need to resolve issues that involve ethical principles on a regular basis. When managing ethical problems, the policy must reflect ethical behavior and promote the caring environments that typify healthcare settings.
5. **Clarity**   A policy needs to be clear in intent and written in a logical manner. A policy specifies its purpose and defines the appropriate methods for attaining that purpose (procedures).

Benefits of Policies and Procedures

A well-conceived policy and procedure manual benefits everyone associated with an organization. Compliance with good patient care standards in a hospital assures the patient the best possible care. Efficiency and safety throughout the organization improve patient services and enhance the quality of work life for employees. A policy is made when responsibility is concisely described and appropriate action for a set of circumstances is outlined. A policy provides general directions to assist the manager in deciding which action to take. The policy is a general rule, not a procedure. Procedures are the detailed directions of implementation of a policy. In other words, policies give direction for action; procedures give step-by-step instructions for carrying out the action.

Preparing the Manual

The language used for writing the manual should be clear and concise. Imperative use of verbs affords the reader only one course of action; for example, write "Complete a Request for Authorization of Overtime form" rather than, "You should complete..."

Mechanical details of the manual that require consideration prior to its issue may include: 1) binding, 2) layout, and 3) indexing—alphabetical, topical or historical.

Check Points

- **Define the audience.** Make the manual easy to read.
- **Include pertinent items.** Assorted policies and procedures unrelated to the service are bulky and confusing.
- **Allow for additions and corrections.** A loose-leaf notebook is preferable for keeping the manual in order and up to date.
- **Use a logical identification system.** Group together policies and procedures that pertain to the same general subject. This manner of assembling the material ensures that the reader sees all that is written on one subject.
- **Aim for clarity with brevity.** A drawing or diagram can facilitate understanding of complicated concepts. Lengthy narratives often go unread.

Policies and Procedures Are Required Characteristics for JCAHO Review

The JCAHO requests that policies and procedures be in place that will assure effective management, safety, equipment performance, communication, and quality control in the radiology department. Written policies and procedures in diagnostic radiology should cover at least the following subjects:

- Who can order a diagnostic radiology procedure and what the mechanism is to request a procedure.
- The appropriateness of diagnostic radiology services requested.
- The proper sequencing and preparations for diagnostic procedures.
- Procedures for patients who require emergency services or are critically ill.
- Informed consent.
- The preparation and administration of intravenous contrast agents.
- Quality control procedures designed to enhance the quality of diagnosis with the minimum risk to patient and personnel.
- Safety procedures for all patient care equipment (See JCAHO standards for "Plant, Technology, and Safety").
- Compliance with all applicable state and federal laws.
- Monitoring of the performance of all diagnostic and therapeutic equipment by a qualified individual.
- Monitoring of doses from diagnostic radiology procedures.
- Adherence to recognized regulations on the safe use of radiation producing equipment.
- Guidelines for protecting personnel and patients from radiation hazards.
- Monitoring hospital staff for exposure to radiation.
- Methods for infection control.
- Employee orientation and safety education.

Organizing the Manual

The scope of the procedure manual is dictated by the size of the department and the energies of the individuals responsible for its preparation. A sample outline is included here and may prove helpful in organizing a manual.

1. Introduction
    a. Purpose of the department of radiology
    b. Mission statement
    c. Objectives of the service
    d. Guest relations
    e. Patient grievance procedures

2. Key personnel
   a. Organization chart (department and hospital)
   b. List of names and addresses of physicians and staff
3. Hours of operation
   a. Hours and days services are available
   b. "Call" schedules and procedures
   c. Radio page numbers
4. Scheduling procedures
   a. Outpatient scheduling
   b. Inpatient scheduling
   c. Examinations available
   d. Order entry system
5. Personnel policies
   a. Job descriptions
   b. Promotion and dismissal
   c. Uniform requirements
   d. Payroll procedures
   e. Shift assignments
   f. Rules of conduct
   g. Career ladders
   h. Orientation
6. The radiology requisition
   a. Flow chart describing requisition procedures
   b. Criteria for judging its completeness
7. Patient preparations
   a. Preparation procedures
   b. Patient education procedures
   c. Patient education materials
   d. Informed consent
8. Safety and handling of patients
   a. Radiation safety rules
   b. Transportation
   c. Lifting and moving
   d. Isolation/infection control techniques
9. Portable radiography
   a. Criteria
   b. Procedures

10. Public safety
    a. Fire
    b. Electrical
    c. Explosion
    d. Hazardous weather
    e. Disaster plan
    f. Bomb scare procedures
    g. Hazardous waste
11. Office procedures
    a. Reception
    b. Clerical functions
    c. Film loan procedures
    d. Transcription
    e. Report delivery/charting
    f. Telephone etiquette
12. Charges
    a. Hospital charges
    b. Professional charges
13. Continuing education
    a. In-service education programs
    b. Institutional staff development
    c. Tuition reimbursement
14. Care of equipment and supplies
    a. Report of malfunction of equipment
    b. Requisitioning of supplies
    c. Inventory control
15. Medical emergency
    a. Management of contrast media reactions
    b. Cardiac arrest/May Day procedures
16. Departmental radiographic routines

Conclusion

The development of policies and procedures requires continual review so the manual is current with the many changes that occur in a radiology department on a daily basis. An auditing process can be used to pinpoint areas of weakness and necessary changes can be made. A good audit consists of (1) a review of all manual contents at least once a year; (2) continual random sampling of operating practice within the department; (3) regular audit reports to the director of the department; and (4) reports to the director of the department of any actions taken on the basis of audit results.

Written policies and procedures bring into focus the relationships among different sections of the department. This focus opens lines of communication and encourages cooperation.

In addition, written policies define the authority of the departmental supervisors, enabling them to confidently make decisions consistent with established operating procedure. This confidence comes from the assured support of their own supervisors.

As the radiology manager assembles policies and procedures, inconsistencies become apparent and can be corrected. This brings about a sense of order. Finally, written policies and procedures related to patient care standards are essential to qualify for payment by some third-party payers and obtain accreditation by regulatory agencies.

The absence of policies and procedures could prevent the department of radiology from meeting JCAHO standards. That possibility may be sufficient motivation for the radiology manager to see that policies and procedures are in order.

3.7   STRATEGIC PLANNING

How many times have you been involved in an informal discussion with peers in your organization and someone jokingly asks, "Where is the man with the plan?" One of the biggest sources of frustration to healthcare managers is attempting to move forward with an idea for service excellence and stumble over obstacles that a manager can't control. The often asked question, "Why doesn't the right hand know what the left hand is doing?" is answered with a well-executed strategic planning process. One healthcare executive prefers to refer to the process of strategic planning as strategic management. Planning, as a function of management, requires that thinking be strategic and long-term, rather than merely reacting to market conditions. The goal of strategic planning is to develop a sustainable competitive advantage over time. From the organization's standpoint, the strategic plan determines where it's going and how it will get there. Planning is a multistep process; it involves the mission statement, data analysis, strategy formulation, developing tactics, implementation and monitoring and evaluation. See figure 3.10.

The Mission Statement

Strategic planning begins with defining the organization's overall goals. Mission statements are difficult to write. They need to accurately portray the purpose of the organization, without being too broad or too specific. Mission statements need flexibility in order to respond to changing needs in the market environment. See figure 3.11. Writing the mission statement for a nonprofit enterprise must balance a duality of purpose. Hospitals need to survive in a deeply financial troubled environment, but at the same time they need to be compassionate and responsive to the needs of the community. Over time, mission statements will change. Increasing specialization and the soaring costs of medical technology and malpractice insurance will cause some hospitals to determine that they can no longer provide comprehensive healthcare to the entire community. The market has become segmented; hospitals are electing to abandon their broad-based acute care provider status in exchange for more focused niche services. New mission statements will reflect those new purposes.

Figure 3.10 Strategic Planning is a Dynamic Process

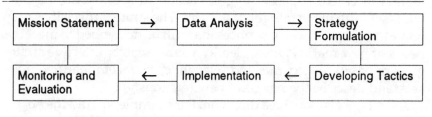

Figure 3.11 Sample Hospital Mission Statement

The hospital is a charitable, not-for-profit organization dedicated to promoting, protecting, and restoring the health of people in the region through the provision of high-quality, cost-effective healthcare services. The hospital is committed to meeting the needs of the region served by caring for those who seek services, regardless of their age, race, sex, religion, nationality, handicaps, or ability to pay.

Data Analysis

The next step in the strategic planning process is data collection—market analysis that will either support or dispute the mission. The data analysis step studies conditions that might affect the organization. The political, legal, regulatory, technologic, economic, and societal environments are carefully surveyed and conclusions drawn are weighed against the organization's purpose. For instance, if the mission statement for a new imaging center states that a broad base of highly technologic services be offered, but market research indicates that competition is keen in this arena, revision of the mission statement might reflect a focused approach to imaging such as women's services. Further support to this change in strategic direction would include a detailed analysis of women's needs and demographics to support these projected needs. Data analysis is an ongoing task, routinely supplying management with information that will nourish the mission and from time to time guide the interpretation of that mission through revisions in programs and services.

Strategy Formulation

Think of strategies as directional action decisions. Armed with market research, strategy suggests action to accomplish the purposes set forth in the mission statement. The strategic decisions may relate to new products or services that will be developed to meet the needs of new markets identified by your research. Effective strategies are based on accurate and relevant data, meet identified markets, and describe the nature of new relationships.

A strategy gives an idea direction. For example, should the hospital develop a freestanding radiation oncology center? Directions to guide this decision will come from numerous sources (e.g., the governing board, planning officials, physicians, etc.). Strategies are directional because they dictate emphasis and force prioritization. A strategy begs action; it creates the expectation that something will happen. Strategies also drive decision making. The decisions are made based on the data collected. Implementation of strategies is dependent upon decision making with action for follow through.

Developing Tactics

Strategy drives tactics. Where strategy concentrates on basic directions, major thrusts, and priorities, tactics carry out the strategy. For example, if the mission statement, borne out by market research data, indicates that the area of sports medicine is underserved by imaging technology, the logical strategy decision might be to initiate MR capability in the affected community. Tactical decisions based on this strategy would relate to actual construction and operations. It is important to note that all tactics do not necessarily lead to implementation of the strategy. Tactics by virtue of their action role in the planning process are subject to trial and error and constant retooling. Tactics give rise to other tactics in the dynamic process of making the strategy a reality.

Implementation

Implementation of tactics becomes operations and usually occurs at lower management levels. Upper management monitors the operations to see how closely the results reflect expectations. These day-to-day operations are shaped by policy—policies set in place to make sure the intent of the original strategy is properly translated into the work of the new program.

Monitoring and Evaluation

A strategic plan should be fluid and include mechanisms for feedback to continually re-evaluate the mission statement and strategies to accomplish that mission. This process of reviewing the written plan is the responsibility of the institutional planning committee. The committee should meet on a quarterly basis to monitor progress towards goals by examining the success of strategies and tactics selected to further those goals.

Guide to Departmental Planning

What Is Planning?

Modern society is in a constant state of change. New discoveries and new technologies are constantly being made that affect the way we think and behave. Rapid and pervasive changes are the hallmark of today's healthcare environment.

Just as other aspects of living change, so do people's healthcare needs change. Health is extremely important; therefore, those of us who provide healthcare services must be ready to meet these ever changing needs. Planning is the tool through which we can know better how to handle the future health requirements of the community that we serve.

The term "planning" covers a wide variety of activities that can range from the simple to the complex. They can involve the solution of current problems facing management to the determination of what actions must be taken to cope with the future. In some cases, planning merely involves translating already made policy decisions into action. Sometimes these are simple; at other times, they are more detailed. In other cases, planning may involve the development of new resources or the construction of new facilities—activites that may span years or require considerable expenditure of funds. Basically, planning is generally recognized as a decision-making process that enables an organization to act today to produce results at some future time.

Planning is also a continuing process. This process does not necessarily result in the preparation of a "plan." At times, it will result in the development of a series of options for future action, some of which may be adopted if certain circumstances or assumptions are realized.

Planning is generally carried out in two separate levels within an organization. One level of planning is carried out by top management whose task involves decision making, guidance of managers, and allocation of resources based on a thorough comprehension of the entire organization. The other aspect of planning is carried out by operational management or the department heads who have two basic charges: 1) managing the direct line functions associated with the hospital's ancillary, support and service departments, and 2) managing resource areas of finance, personnel, information, inventory, etc. within their departments.

The Planning Process

Planning is a responsibility shared by staff at all levels within the organization. The governing board and administration do not dictate to each department what its goals should be. Instead, departments are responsible for examining their own needs and the needs of patients they serve and from that perspective, developing goals and strategies to suit the department. Administration does provide overall direction to planning by setting broad goals that outline the basic purpose of the institution and by approving all departmental goals and strategies. Otherwise, departments are permitted much freedom in the planning process.

Steps in the Planning Process

Planning is an orderly process that follows a series of steps which, when fully accomplished, will result in an overall planning document. This document, known as the Strategic Plan, will contain a mission statement and the direction it will take in the near future.

The Strategic Plan will then be interpreted and translated into short-range (annual) operating plans by the manager. The steps below present the sequence of events that will occur in the planning process:

1. The governing board, upon recommendation of the Institutional Strategic Planning Committee, will adopt a Strategic Plan that will describe the desired future of the organization.
2. Department heads and supervisors will attend a planning orientation to learn details of the planning process. The orientation will describe what is involved in planning, and what should be considered in developing departmental goals, strategies, tactics, and budget. During the session, goals, strategies, and budget assumptions for the coming year will be distributed

and discussed, emphasizing that these should only form the frame of reference in which departmental goals, the strategies necessary to accomplish those goals, and budgets are prepared.

3. A deadline will be set by which departmental goals and strategies must be complete. Each department may use any management style for determining goals. However, department heads are encouraged to involve other members of their staff as much as possible in planning. This broadens the base of support for the departmental goals, increases employees' feelings of involvement, and generates a wider variety of ideas for potential goals and strategies.

4. The goals and strategies are reviewed by the director of planning and forwarded to administration. Departments will then be asked to make corrections if any problems are found. Administration will review the goals and strategies affecting more than one department or the hospital as a whole.

5. When all departmental goals have been approved in administration, they will be forwarded, along with the departmental budget, to the Budget Committee for its review. Should the Budget Committee's decision affect the ability of a department to carry out its stated goals and strategies, those affected goals and strategies will be rewritten by the department, and the approval process is repeated for those revised goals and strategies.

6. The significance of planning is diminished if the goals and objectives are put on the shelf and never implemented. Therefore, the final stage of planning must be conducted. This stage is evaluation. Evaluation is an opportunity to measure accomplishments and to determine what progress the department has made and what further action is necessary. Evaluation is part of an overall effectiveness measuring system for the organization.

Setting Department Goals

Writing meaningful goals and strategies does require careful thought, preparation, and creativity. An excellent way to facilitate this process is to exchange ideas with other members of your staff and other department heads.

Deciding what goals and strategies the department should carry out in the coming years will begin with an understanding of current practices. This is done by examining four major areas: (Figure 3.12 provides a worksheet that may be used for this purpose).

1. What is the department's basic reason or purpose for existing and is it fulfilling that purpose? If not, what changes are needed to meet its purpose?
2. What are the department's major strengths (e.g., resources, such as staff, equipment and facilities), what can be accomplished with these resources, and what additional resources are required?
3. What are the department's major weaknesses? What obstacles exist that should be removed to allow optimum functioning of the department?
4. What trends exist in the key areas of the department listed below?
    a. The department's volume—the output or number of patients served.
    b. The quality of services provided including the number of errors, patient satisfaction, etc.
    c. The department's financial condition.
    d. The department's productivity and efficiency with which it delivers services.
    e. The growth of new services provided through the department.

By looking closely at these trends, it should be possible to determine where departmental activities can be improved or where problems exist that need to be solved.

In developing goals and strategies, a department may also examine the needs in the community/services area and evaluate whether it can provide services to meet those needs. However, reference should be made to the strategic plan for an indication of the economic and political trends that could affect service delivery and community health needs.

In summary, the method of developing department goals and strategies focuses on an assessment of what the department currently does and then determines what it can do in the future.

Figure 3.12 Departmental Assessment Worksheet

Directions: This worksheet is designed to assist departments in determining areas
     where improvements are needed. It is for your internal use only and is not to
     be submitted with goals statements.

1. What is the department's basic purpose (reason for being)?
2. What are the department's most important activities?
     a)
     b)
     c)
     d)
     e)
3. Evaluate each of the above activities (more than satisfied, acceptable, below
     minimal expectations) in terms of a) quality of service/care being provided,
     b) efficiency/productivity of service delivery, c) degree to which budget is met,
     and other criteria you may want to use.
4. What are the major weaknesses/problems that may prevent the department
     from fulfilling its purpose or carrying out its major activities?
     a)
     b)
     c)
     d)
     e)
5. What actions are needed to correct the above noted weaknesses?
     a)
     b)
     c)
     d)
     e)
6. List new programs, innovative ideas for service delivery, possible areas of
     expanded services, etc. that the department would like to see implemented
     (may not necessarily be related to problems noted above).
     a)
     b)
     c)
     d)

Writing Departmental Goals

Once a goal is determined, it is necessary to choose the proper way
to phrase it. A goal should be stated clearly so that other people (e.g.,
nonprofessionals) can read and understand its intent. The following
rules for writing goals may be helpful:

1. A goal is a statement of a result that you want to achieve.

2. A goal should start with the word "to" followed by an action verb, since a goal can only be achieved as a result of some action you take. (Please refer to Appendix A.)
3. A goal should state only "what" is to be accomplished and not "how" or "why."
4. A goal should be something you can measure or observe so you (or someone else) would easily know when it has been accomplished (e.g., "to increase outpatient visits by 25 percent" is measurable).
5. Goals should not comprise a "laundry list" of staff or equipment desired (e.g., "to purchase a digital vascular imaging system" is not an acceptable goal by itself).

Determining Department Strategies

After goals have been written, a decision must then be made as to how the goals will be achieved. There are several different ways that are better than others. Below is a list of guidelines to follow in determining what strategies and tactics best lead to implementation of the goal:

1. List several different strategies through which the goal could be implemented. Determine the resources that would be required for each tactic (new staff, new equipment, new facilities, improved productivity/efficiency, etc.) and which tactics appear to have the greatest likelihood of successfully achieving the goal. Based on this analysis, select the most efficient and effective series of tactics for the strategies necessary to attain the goal.
2. Decide who in the department should be responsible for seeing that a strategy is carried out. Implementation of strategies, and thus the goal, is best attained when an individual is assigned the task of supervising the tactic steps.
3. Determine a deadline when the strategy is to be completed or when it is to be fully operational if it represents an ongoing service.*

---

*"The Guide to Department Planning" was contributed by Charles H. Meehan of Columbia, S.C.

Change Is the Future

Change has characterized healthcare in the last three decades, and the 1990s are expected to bring more of the same. According to Dale Collins, President and CEO of the Baptist Health System of East Tennessee:

- The 1960s was a period of access to healthcare for everyone, and a period of phenomenal growth and attention to patient care.
- In the 1970s healthcare spending continued and concerns grew about unbridled expansion and duplication of services.
- The 1980s was a period of federal deficits and a time of growth in managed care. Healthcare costs became a major burden and the fastest growing segment of the federal budget.
- The 1990s will be a time of challenge, of rising anger about healthcare costs, of a desire to increase quality at reduced costs, and of a shift of burden on paying for access to healthcare to providers.

"Unstable," "unpredictable," "chaotic," and "unmanageable" are what managers think about the world of healthcare they face. It is obvious that change is here to stay; there will be no return to the "good old days" or "the way we used to do it." Therefore, management structures that worked in the past cannot be relied on to work in the future. Strategically, we need change in our organizations to adapt and to evolve with the future. As managers we need to become adept at analyzing dynamic market conditions and implementing the strategies necessary for survival. As a radiology manager, be proactive and an initiator in managing this change process through the strategic planning process.

Appendix A

A List of Verbs Useful in Writing Department Strategies

Fact Finding:

analyze	evaluate	institute	observe	survey
audit	examine	inspect	review	validate
calculate	experiment	interview	score	

| check | gather | inventory | search |
| compute | identify | investigate | study |

Planning and Scheduling:

arrange	control	layout	register
assemble	describe	organize	schedule
assign	determine	plan	stock
budget	estimate	prepare	store
catalog	forecast	provide	submit
compile	formulate	regulate	supply

Influencing and/or Establishing Standards:

adopt	decide	establish	present
approve	design	initiate	recommend
classify	determine	modify	set
construct	develop	organize	specify
create	devise	prescribe	

Relationships:

accept	contribute	furnish	receive
advise	cooperate	guide	select
approve	coordinate	install	sell
assist	counsel	interpret	send
attend	deliver	maintain	translate
commit	demonstrate	negotiate	transmit
confer	exchange	participate	tutor
consolidate	expedite	procure	utilize
contract	explain	provide	
facilitate	purchase		

Conducting or Doing:

act	disseminate	lecture	proofread
administer	draft	maintain	repair
brief	edit	manage	research
carry out	execute	monitor	review
conduct	exercise	operate	staff
control	fabricate	orient	supervise
coordinate	file	perform	teach
demonstrate	implement	process	transport
direct	instruct	program	write

3.8   Facility Planning

Yesterday a radiology manager, today a construction project coordinator! The tasks of starting new services or upgrading old ones frequently involves the matching of high technology with construction. A building program with major construction has many pitfalls. The coordination of these many details that must fall into place is one of the most complex and treacherous tasks a manager can face. Here are just some errors that could have been prevented with better preconstruction planning.

- A West Coast hospital wanted to construct a 20,000 square foot free-standing imaging center to include 20 imaging examination rooms. The architect was not given specific information on how the rooms would be used and, with limited healthcare experience, assumed all the rooms would be an equal size.
- A radiographic/fluoroscopic room so small that the entrance door bumped the table and could not be opened fully to allow passage of a wheelchair or stretcher.
- A darkroom without plumbing.
- A lavatory with a specimen pass-through box where the door to the pass-through was obstructed from opening by the tank on the toilet.
- Installation of an R/F table that tilts the patient out of the view of the operator's booth.
- Inability to park an image intensifier in a location that would not collide with the examination table.
- Failure to reinforce floors to support the additional weight of equipment such as MR.
- Overlooked the need for piped in medical gases in a special procedures room.

The Importance of Planning

Construction planning entails more than determining optimum patient throughput for an imaging center or hospital radiology department. It is step-by-step analysis of the function and location of each detail of the building program. You will consider every piece of equipment, every lighting switch, every piece of door hardware, every plumbing fixture, and every texture and finish of the interiors. Persons unfamiliar with the construction process are easily over-whelmed by the number of decisions that are made. Compounding an already fragile situation is the occasional architect who does not know healthcare. Even design firms with hospital experience will still rely on the clinical and technical skills of the proposed facility's users. A successful design will depend upon cooperation from both the architect and the hospital's design team. Patrick B. Davis, Jr., AIA of Sarasota, Florida, says that most hospitals have an architectural firm they use on an ongoing basis for projects. Using the same architectural firm for most hospitals is a matter of convenience and practicality. If you're looking for a new architectural firm, Davis suggests that firms should offer the following:

- Previous successful experience.
- Previous working relationship with facility or administration.
- Understanding of program.
- Knowledge of local building codes.
- Knowledge of site.
- Demonstration of sensitivity to provide high quality environments.
- Commitment to meet budget and schedule.
- Know who will actually do the work.
- Technical expertise.

Once the architect is hired and the project is designed, specified, and bid out, you will select a contractor to build your dream depart-ment. The capabilities of that contractor will determine whether you have a free-flowing project where everything fits together nicely or whether you have a disaster on your hands. Take this example of a California hospital that built an ambulatory care center with an MR suite. It seemed that every design contingency was covered; namely, lead shielding, floor structure reinforcement, and upgraded electri-cal and mechanical services. The contractor worked with two archi-tects, two subcontractors, a consultant, and a physicist. In the elev-enth hour, it was discovered that computer cables adjacent to the MR gantry room would distort images. No one would accept responsi-bility for this design flaw. This is a classic case of "segmented accountability." To avoid it, choose the contractor with the ability to do the whole job and be responsible for the continuity of the project. James Zampetti of Long Beach, California, suggests that the one contractor selected should be able to manage every aspect of the project to include:

1. Planning.
2. Design.
3. Engineering.
4. Financing.
5. Site Preparation.
6. Permit Compliance.
7. Construction.
8. Inspection.
9. Landscaping.

Bud W. Hunton, MA, RT(R) of Dayton, Ohio, says that whether you're installing a major piece of equipment, building new offices or dressing rooms, or completely revamping a department, a basic planning process should be followed to optimize efficiency, expedite the project, and contain costs. Hunton suggests a project check off sheet could include the items listed here:

- Permits or licenses.
- Structural requirements.
- Environmental support.
- Air-conditioning and heating.
- Plumbing and electrical specifications.
- Interior finishes, counters, floor and wall coverings.
- Ventilation.
- Masonry, tile, trims.
- Safety requirements.
- Forms to fill out.
- Furnishings.

Common Design Mistakes in Imaging

Failing to Be Customer Oriented

Design imaging service areas around customer needs. Just as you know when you have arrived at a McDonald's Restaurant by passing those golden arches, so should registration and reception be unmistakable in the radiology department. Arrange the registration function in a private setting to obtain confidential and usually sensitive information in a professional manner. The reception area should be furnished with comfortable but sturdy seating, and it should be arranged in a manner that affords privacy. Single seating is preferred in "waiting rooms" because a person who is unaccompanied will rarely sit with a stranger on a 2 or 3 seat sofa. Single seating is much more flexible and efficient to use and may be clustered in smaller private groupings. A large rectangular room will be more efficient by holding more patients, but an L- or T-shaped room will allow more privacy by using smaller seating arrangements in clusters.

Keeping customer satisfaction in mind, don't repeat the mistakes made in the past for patient changing areas. Hospital radiology departments used to predominantly serve an inpatient population, so changing cubicles for outpatients were often a neglected area. In the past, it was common practice to centralize changing cubicles in one location in the department, thus forcing scantily gowned patients to walk long distances to examining rooms. Modern imaging department design incorporates decentralized changing cubicles and sub-waiting areas that open directly into the various procedure rooms. An efficient way to arrange changing cubicles is to plan for three changing cubicles per procedure room and to arrange the design of the procedure rooms so that a group of three procedure rooms would have up to nine changing cubicles with one toilet facility. In a fluoroscopy area, direct access to toilet facilities should be from the procedure room and there should be always two toilet rooms per fluoroscopy room.

With the current shift of emphasis on outpatient imaging services, don't lose sight of the importance of maintaining dignity for inpatients as well. There has been a proliferation of outpatient imaging centers in this country in the last decade; however, most hospital radiology departments still cater to both an inpatient and outpatient population. Inpatients require special considerations as well. Maintaining the dignity and confidentiality of inpatients is another primary concern that must be addressed by efficient department design. When working with a program that calls for integration of the radiology department into the general hospital, a separate entrance for inpatients will avoid transporting nonambulatory patients through public waiting rooms. Most radiology managers are familiar with single-corridor designed x-ray departments where inpatients are parked outside the examination room awaiting their turn. A more customer-friendly design allows for inpatient holding rooms that will provide monitoring of these patients and maintain their privacy. These inpatient holding areas can also double as recovery rooms following invasive procedures. See figure 3.13 for some tips in MRI planning.

Planning for Adequate Support Space

Adequate space for support functions, such as administrative offices, clerical areas, staff facilities and storage, is an area often underemphasized in the planning of imaging departments. Planners

Figure 3.13   Common Design Flaws in Planning a new MRI Facility*

What may seem like a small annoyance or inconvenience in the planning stage of a new facility can often snowball into a major problem during construction. These are some areas to check for possible design flaws:

Window positioning. A common error is placing the window too far above the control console. It's important to make sure the technologist can simultaneously operate the equipment and see into the examination room. In one facility, someone tapped the technologist on the shoulder while she was monitoring an MRI procedure, breaking her concentration. She turned toward the interloper and asked in effect, "Will you please get out of here?" It turned out to be the patient, who had wiggled out of the magnet, changed clothes, and was stopping by to let the technologist know of his premature departure.

Communications. Where should the telephones be placed? What kind of intercom system should you have? Will it be easy to operate? What rooms should you link into the system? Planning an efficient communications system is extremely important.

Instrumentation. Instruments should be wrapped comfortably around the operator's station so as to provide easy access and viewing. And make sure there is adequate lighting with no glare on the computer screen.

Storage. Often this is an afterthought, but it shouldn't be. Insufficient or inconvenient storage areas—cabinets, shelves, closets—can cost you dearly in terms of time, energy, and irritation. No one should have to walk far or climb on a step stool to retrieve commonly used items. Although radiology department personnel often complain about not having *enough* storage space, in most cases what they really mean is that they don't have properly designed storage areas in the right locations. Often storage areas in MRI units look as if they were modeled after kitchen cabinets, with space allotted for pots, pans, and dishes rather than for the supplies they use.

---

* Adapted from: Planning a new MRI Facility: Avoiding Common Mistakes. *Imaging Economics.* Vol. 1, No. 3, 1992.

refer to the support spaces as "soft areas," and the tendency by hospital managers is to encroach upon these soft areas to make space for technology. Ask any radiology manager if he has adequate filing space and then brace yourself for a horror story about the necessity for off-site film storage and a saga of lost film jackets. Predicting how much administrative space will be necessary in order to manage the facility into the future is also a difficult task that is weighed against both present and anticipated technologic requirements. The effects of future growth will also impact on staff facilities such as locker rooms and lounges. These spaces are often the only places that staff members without offices have to retreat for relief from the work environment.

As mentioned earlier, records storage is every radiology manager's personal nightmare. Most radiology departments like to keep two to three years of x-ray film within an easily retrievable distance. Movable film file systems, although expensive, will substantially increase the storage capacity of a file area. It is important to take into consideration that when fully loaded these movable filing systems will weigh between 250 and 300 pounds per square foot of floor space.

Finding space for other kinds of storage will also be necessary. In order to keep procedure rooms and areas visible to the public free of clutter, a storage area large enough to meet the requirements of predicted examination volumes should be located close at hand. In addition, plan for linens, exchange carts, the parking of portable x-ray equipment, and a place to keep wheelchairs and stretchers when not in use. See figure 3.14 for 10 common errors to avoid while planning new space.

Figure 3.14 10 Common Errors to Avoid

- Lack of pre-programming and site planning
- Disregard for activity zones and traffic flow
- Inappropriate lighting
- Ineffective communications equipment
- Inadequate storage and staff areas
- Undersized patient waiting & holding areas
- Minimal square footage in exam and control areas
- Remote and inadequate archival film storage
- Disregard for visual esthetics
- Poor attention to "details"

From: Managing Successful Radiology Projects, an RSNA '92 presentation by Rostenberg, B., Campbell, J., and Stein, M. Chicago, Ill.

Designing for Maximum Workflow

Traffic patterns are a main consideration in developing the plan, which must ensure that radiology personnel will function at peak efficiency. Patient flow within the department is a prime consideration. The patient should be kept waiting as little as possible from the time of reception through the final quality review process and dismissal. Traffic patterns produced by technical personnel and radiologists are the next most important considerations. Minimizing the number of steps necessary for personnel to complete their tasks will maximize efficiency. Typical radiographer activity is traced in the flow chart in figure 3.15.

The radiologist's time is divided between examining patients, consultation, and film interpretation. A flow chart of daily activity for a radiologist is shown in figure 3.16. Radiologists should have private offices within easy access of the reading and consultation area.

A good configuration for the radiology department is some variation from a basic square or deep rectangle. Less desirable configurations may be found in examples of the single-corridor design and wing-type arrangements. The shape of the department determines traffic patterns; therefore, design considerations that make the radiology department a pleasant and efficient work area are key issues.

Small radiology departments are often a **single-corridor design**. This design can be functional when the single corridor is dead-ended, but often the department lies on either side of a corridor continuous with other hospital traffic. Passing the radiology department on the way to another area may not pose a problem for the traveler, but it can be disruptive to the radiology department. A single-corridor plan works best when only radiology traffic is allowed, and when patients are received on one end and are exited at the other end. A single-corridor concept is illustrated in figure 3.17.

The **two-corridor design** is simple to conceptualize; it is also known as the "sandwich design." Examining rooms and dark rooms are between support areas, off corridors on either side. One corridor (at the back) becomes a staff working area, and the corridor in the front is for patient traffic. Figure 3.18 illustrates the two-corridor

Figure 3.15 Radiographer Activity Depicted as a Circular Path

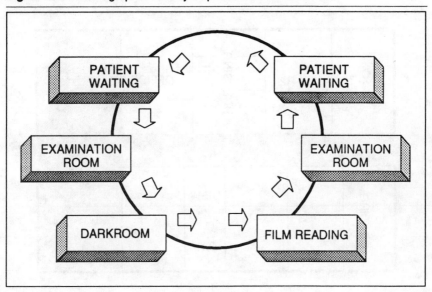

Figure 3.16 Flow Chart of Radiologist Activity

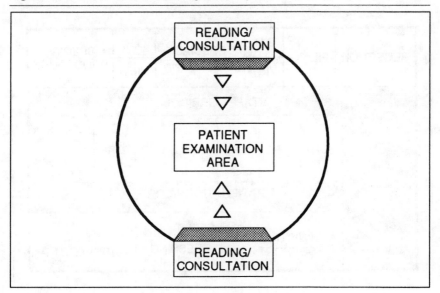

Figure 3.17   Single-Corridor Plan

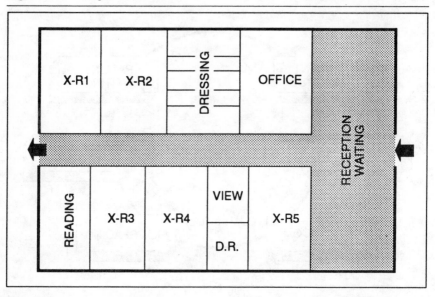

Figure 3.18   Two-Corridor Design

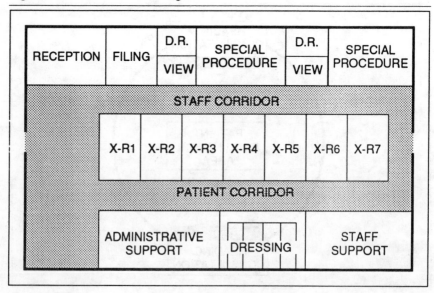

design and some of its shortcomings, which are a result of distance. Communication from one end to the other and dispersed film handling make it diffcult to monitor quality control. The amount of walking that personnel must do from one location to another is also counterproductive.

Separate sections identified by the type of radiologic examination performed in them may be arranged in a **wing design** clustered around a central area. These areas are sometimes described as pods and may be associated with urology, gastrointestinal procedures, special procedures, routine radiographic studies, or pediatrics. Each wing identifies with a central control area where the administration of the department is conducted. (See Figure 3.19)

The **mirror-design** concept of radiology department layout shares the basic ideas of the wing design. The configuration of the department may be semicircular with a central area at the front of the half-circle. Another half-circle, a mirror image in construction, faces the other side of the central area. (See Figure 3.20)

With this design, initial construction of the radiology department can be accomplished, and the mirror image may be completed later. Both sides of the design will eventually form one coherent department. The main benefit of this concept is that projected expansion will allow an orderly progression toward one large, well-functioning area (see Figure 3.21).

The **central-core** design is a square or rectangular area. The core, or center, is formed by one activity and surrounded by another. For example, the center could be used for film processing and sorting, and the area around it could consist of examining rooms. Figure 3.22 represents the concept of the central-core design with the examining rooms along the outside walls of the core.

Planning for Efficient Work Flow

Each patient in the radiology department generates a permanent medical record to be maintained by the department. The actual radiographs are part of this record, along with the official report and radiograph envelope. The patient record begins at the front desk where the

Figure 3.19 Wing Design Concept

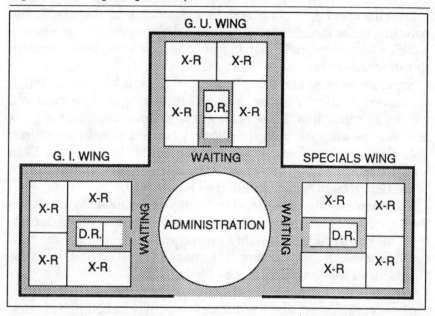

Figure 3.20 Mirror-Design Concept

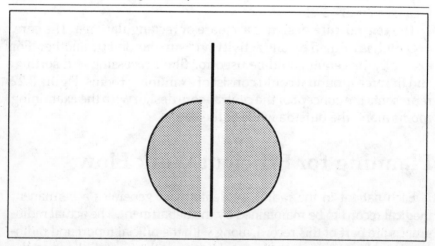

Figure 3.21 Mirror-Design Plan

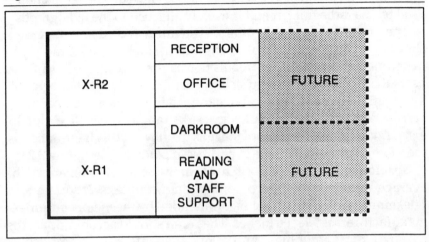

Figure 3.22 Central-Core Design

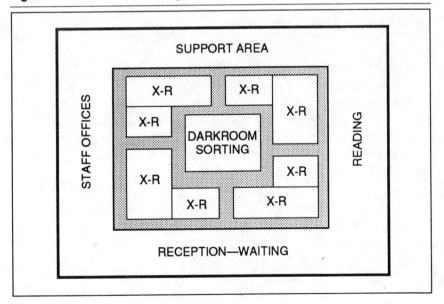

requisition for radiology services is first reviewed. The requisition is used by the radiographer and is usually attached to the radiographs.

The importance of designing a system for **records management** should be emphasized in planning discussions. In most radiology departments, the radiology requisition is the official document that bears the signature of the physician ordering the study. Demographic information and clinical indications are usually found on this document, and these facts are used by radiology clerks, radiographers, and radiologists. A logical approach to managing the flow of this information is, therefore, an important issue to address in planning. See figure 3.23.

Spaciousness and ease of movement are key elements. The average radiographic-fluoroscopic room occupies 350 square feet. The minimum ceiling height recommended by the major equipment manufacturers is 9 feet 6 inches. The room should accommodate the required x-ray equipment and allow adequate import and export space for beds and stretchers. The generator is usually found in one corner of the room. A generator room that may be shared by a number of examining rooms can be built, or the generator can be placed in an

Figure 3.23   Records Management

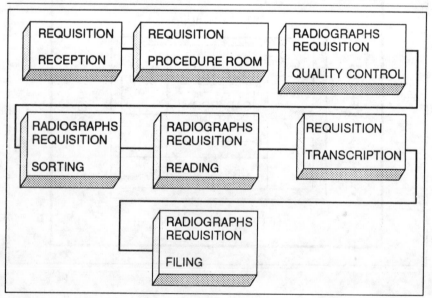

interfloor space, above or below the examining room. A typical design for a radiographic-fluoroscopic room is illustrated in figure 3.24.

Twenty-five square feet is the minimum size for the **control area**. It should allow for the observation of the patient when the table is in the upright position, and the viewing window should be large enough for radiographers of any stature to view the room. Verbal and visual contact with the patient is essential; a speak-through vent or intercom system can be used for this purpose. The control area should be designed so that protection from the primary beam is accomplished without a door, which could interfere with quick access to the patient during emergencies.

Minimal travel to the **darkroom** is a prime consideration for the radiographer. Processing in radiology departments falls into two categories: centralized and distributed. The management of film processing through the centralized method employs one large darkroom area in a convenient location. One darkroom location centralizes quality control. It also means that a breakdown in the darkroom will cause a work stoppage in the whole department.

Figure 3.24 Simple Radiographic/Fluoroscopic Design

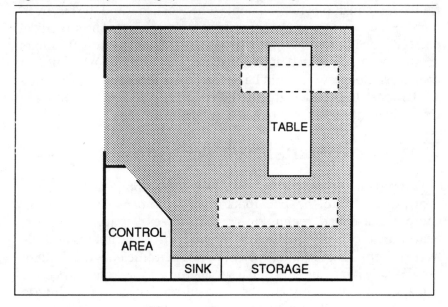

The distributed method of film processing is commonly found in new radiology departments. Radiographic rooms are clustered around a small processing area, and the department may contain two or more of these distributed film processing centers. Despite the kind of arrangements selected for the department, the essential parts of the darkroom remain the same. As daylight film management systems gain popularity, design considerations for radiographic processing will change. Nonetheless darkroom facilities will remain a department fixture for the foreseeable future.

Film reading functions can be centralized or distributed. In a small radiology department, one radiologist would likely have a combined office and reading area. The office should be large enough to accommodate group viewing. When two or more radiologists work together, a central reading area is a definite advantage over distributed reading areas. The reading room should allow 80 square feet for each reading station. Advantages of a central reading area include the following: 1) There is easy access to radiologists for consultation; 2) radiologists are able to confer on difficult cases; and 3) most of the film jackets will be found in one area, making it easier for retrieving and refiling film jackets.

The design of the radiology department should carefully account for the relationship between people who work in it and the **environment of the work place**. Care should be taken to see that no structural obstructions interfere with the functions of the department. Pillars should be incorporated into the design of the department and changes in floor level should be avoided. Air should be conditioned at a temperature comfortable for both staff and patients. Lighting in the patient care areas must be of adjustable intensity.

Plan for Expansion Up Front

Equipment manufacturers are designing equipment that fits in nearly two-thirds of the space that former equipment needed. Newer computer assisted technologies require less space; therefore, healthcare architects are downsizing imaging departments and delivering tight designs that sacrifice operational efficiency and patient flow. Where it may be true that a smaller procedure room is needed to install modern equipment, the room still needs to be large enough to maneuver about with a stretcher and any number of gadgets that may be attached to a critically ill patient. The room must be large enough to allow staff adequate space to reach all sides of the imaging equipment without being an acrobat. Figure 3.25 suggests some procedure room sizes for various types of equipment. The square footage stated is for the procedure room only; use a factor of 30 percent in planning for other functions around the procedure room such as corridors, dressing rooms, toilets, control rooms. Design procedure rooms for flexibility in the future. Try not to design the room around a piece of equipment; instead, use universal style designs for electrical chases and overhead suspensions that will accommodate many manufacturers' equipment.

Keeping up with technology makes the radiology department the most frequently modified space in the hospital. The ability to expand or renovate without completely closing down operations is a must for future development.

In the past, radiology has usually been located in the basement or the first floor of the hospital. Often nestled between major functions such as surgery and the emergency room, it was thought that having radiology adjacent to these functions was efficient. Although that may still be true, the expandability of the radiology department is hampered by the location of its neighbors. If the opportunity exists to place your imaging facility anywhere in the building, then look for neighbors that will be in soft space; namely, space that is easily redesigned for another purpose. It is much easier to encroach upon conference rooms and offices when the time comes for radiology to expand. A final suggestion about location would be to locate the radiology department against an outside wall of the building, so when all of the soft space located on the inside of the building is consumed, expansion is still possible by moving outward.

Figure 3.25 Recommended Radiology Procedure Room Sizes

Chest Room	125 Square Feet
General Radiographic Room	300 Square Feet
R/F Room	350 Square Feet
Radiographic/Tomographic	300 Square Feet
Mammography	150 Square Feet
Ultrasound Room	65 Square Feet
CT Scan Room	275 Square Feet
Special Procedures Room	600 Square Feet
MR Gantry Room	600 Square Feet

Conceptual Design Models*

User wants are translated into planning criteria for use in determining the physical design of an imaging facility. Although no two imaging centers are identical in plan or design, most new facilities can be categorized into four basic conceptual design models: freestanding, medical mall component, hospital-attached, and hospital-integrated.

Freestanding

A freestanding facility is an independent structure that houses only diagnostic imaging services. This facility may be located on a dedicated site or as part of a larger medical campus. A unique feature of this model allows the overall building form to be determined based on functional needs rather than on designing the space to fit within an existing area with defined physical parameters. For example, a traditional centralized imaging suite design with procedure rooms clustered around a central film processing core will have a different building floor plan than a design where procedure rooms and processing areas are decentralized throughout the department. In a freestanding facility, operational concepts are able to dictate facility design. (See Figure 3.26)

Medical Mall Component

The medical mall concept was developed to provide outpatient diagnostic and treatment services as an alternative to a hospital-based location. Imaging services—along with laboratory, pharmacy services, and private physician offices—are key components of the medical mall concept.

Providing these services outside of the traditional hospital setting also has a financial benefit—a lower construction cost. Medical malls (as well as freestanding buildings) are not subject to the same stringent construction and building code requirements that hospitals must follow, which results in outpatient facilities being built at a lower construction cost per square foot. (See Figure 3.27)

---

*This section on conceptual design originally appeared in Keenan, L. A. and Goldman, E. F. "Positive Imaging: Design as Marketing Tool in Diagnostic Centers." *Administrative Radiology.* 8(2): 39-40, 1989. Used with permission of the publisher.

Figure 3.26 Operational Concepts in a Freestanding Facility

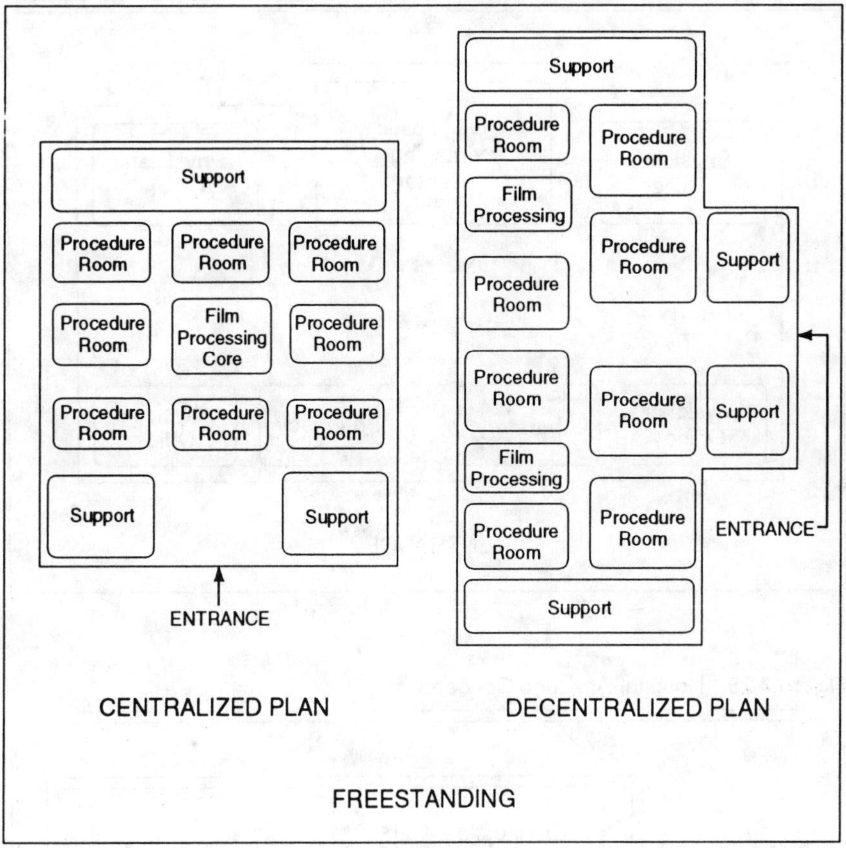

CENTRALIZED PLAN   DECENTRALIZED PLAN

FREESTANDING

Hospital-Attached

Under this model, a diagnostic imaging center is designed as an independent component of a hospital building. Maintaining a clear-cut physical separation between the imaging center (i.e., patient registration, waiting rooms, changing rooms, procedure rooms, and staff work areas) distinctly separate from the inpatient radiology department and other hospital services is a key design element.

The outpatient imaging center may or may not have a dedicated entrance from the outside. However, a dedicated entrance is preferable because it does not require a patient to walk through unrelated hospital areas and thereby reinforces the outpatient environment. (See Figure 3.28)

Figure 3.27   Medical Mall Concept

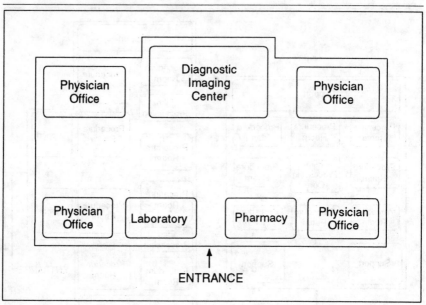

Figure 3.28   Hospital-Attached Concept

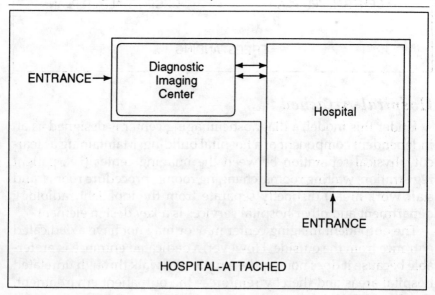

Hospital-Integrated

An outpatient-oriented imaging service may be integrated into a traditional hospital-based radiology setting. This concept encourages maximum utilization, while reducing duplication of costly radiological equipment, since all patient procedures are performed in a centralized location. An important design concept in this model consists of separating outpatients from inpatient and emergency patients within the department. A separate entrance, preferably direct from the outside, and support areas dedicated for outpatient use (i.e., patient registration, waiting room, changing rooms, toilet facilities) physically separated from inpatient support area (i.e., receiving, stretcher and wheelchair holding) are essential design features that are required to provide a distinct outpatient-oriented imaging service.

Operational advantages to this model and the hospital-attached model are that support services provided in a hospital setting may serve the outpatient-oriented imaging service. Hospital-based computerized admission systems, housekeeping and maintenance services, and quick access to medical backup in the event of a patient code are just some of the services available for shared support. (See Figure 3.29)

Figure 3.29 Hospital-Shared Concept

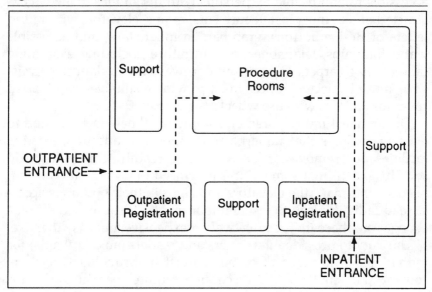

Clearly, there are facility considerations important to the marketing of diagnostic imaging centers. Such considerations are based on identification of user segments and their wants, which, when completed, result in the general design criteria of accessibility, privacy/comfort/security, throughput, turnaround time, comprehensiveness, and cost. The freestanding design model conceptually meets these criteria the best, followed by the medical mall and hospital-attached models. Specific facility plans will, of course, have developmental constraints to them, which may or may not result in the same model evaluation. Marketing staff are often left out of facility development processes. Regardless of who is involved, a marketing orientation is required for a positive image to be projected.

How does the ADA affect the design and construction of medical offices?*

In the past, patients with mobility impairments and other physical disabilities had difficulty gaining access to care because physicians' offices were not designed to accommodate such patients. The new law requires that all places of public accommodation be made readily accessible to and usable by persons with disabilities. Newly constructed offices must install curb cuts, ramps, elevators with raised letters or Braille buttons, grab bars in toilet stalls, and accessible water fountains, telephones, and furniture, including examining tables. Shag carpets and narrow doorways are no longer permissible, and physicians' offices must provide a suitable examination room for patients who use wheelchairs.

The architectural requirements apply to all new facilities and to existing facilities that undergo renovations. In addition, existing facilities must remove barriers where it is "readily achievable" to do so. This means that some offices may need to install ramps where needed, and make the elevators and signs in their buildings accessible to individuals with visual impairments. "Readily achievable" changes are those that are relatively inexpensive and easy to make.

The duty to provide interpreters and readers (auxiliary aids) for individuals who are deaf or blind must be provided where the content and length of the discussion require them in order for

---

*Matson, Holleman, Nosek and Wilkinson. *The Journal of Family Practice*. 36(2): 204-205, 1993.

"effective communication" to be achieved. In other situations "effective communication" may be achieved through the use of computer terminals or a notepad and paper. These auxiliary aids must be provided unless the physician's office can demonstrate that it would impose an undue burden requiring significant difficulty or expense.

Conclusion

The functions of medical imaging will continue to change with advances in technology; these changes will dictate that imaging facilities will continue to be expanded and renovated to reflect the needs of an increasingly sophisticated and competitive market. One can only hope that we will not create new facilities and inherit the same problems. Planning prior to construction and continuous inspection during the building phase will avoid expensive pitfalls. Construction planning involves decisions about technology and building materials and the facilities' overall appearance. Clearly, there are facility considerations that will be based on marketing information about users and their wants. Understanding the needs of the populations served will result in design criteria that assures ease of access, security, and effectiveness.

A reconciliation of form and function will promote longevity of the use of the building and spaces that are operationaly effective. The approach is simply one of farsightedness and flexibility and of a firm understanding of users' requirements and preferences. The diagram on the following page very nicely describes the architectural process in medical terms.

Appendix A

Top 25 Most Frequently Performed Radiology Procedures*

1. CT scan of head
2. Diagnostic ultrasound of heart
3. Routine chest x-ray
4. CT scan of abdomen
5. Diagnostic ultrasound of abdomen

---

*Adapted from *Healthweek—Desktop Resource*. September 24, 1990, from a report prepared by Healthcare Knowledge Systems (CPHA). Ann Arbor, MI.

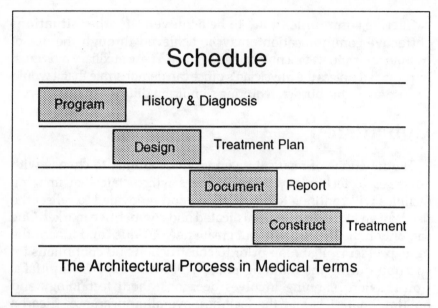

Schedule

Program	History & Diagnosis
Design	Treatment Plan
Document	Report
Construct	Treatment

The Architectural Process in Medical Terms

From: Managing Successful Radiology Projects an RSNA '92 presentation by Rostenberg, B., Campbell, J. and Stein, M., Chicago, Ill.

6. Isotope vascular scan
7. Other CT scan
8. Isotope bone scan
9. Diagnostic ultrasound of digestive tract
10. Isotope pulmonary scan
11. Abdominal x-ray
12. Lower GI series
13. Chest x-ray
14. Diagnostic ultrasound of head and neck
15. Diagnostic ultrasound of urinary tract
16. Pregnancy ultrasound
17. Diagnostic ultrasound NEC
18. CT scan of thorax
19. Isotope liver scan
20. Diagnostic vascular ultrasound
21. Skeletal x-ray of pelvis and hip
22. X-ray of urinary system
23. Small bowel series
24. Lumbrosacral spine x-ray
25. Upper GI with barium

Appendix B

Planning Suggestions for Ultrasound, Nuclear Medicine, CT and MRI Functions*

Ultrasound or Nuclear Medicine Suite Layout

• Floor space of 55 to 65 square feet and a standard ceiling height of 12 feet are adequate for each room.
• Two patient berths per room will facilitate patient throughput.
• Dedicated wall outlets behind each machine will avoid having the power cables crossing the floor and will promote safety.
• Ample storage space to reduce clutter.
• Wall-hung stainless steel sink for infection control and medicine preparation.
• Room should be maintained at a constant 75 degrees Fahrenheit. Remember, the machines produce sufficient heat to necessitate cooling at a rate in excess of 18,000 BTUs per hour.

CT Suite Layout

• The procedure room should be at least 276 square feet to accommodate the gantry table.
  — Interface cables to the various components of the system should be accommodated in prefabricated trough conduits mounted beneath the floor.
  — Fluorescent and incandescent lighting recessed in ceiling for safety.
  — Ample storage space should be planned for linen, contrast media, and intravenous supplies.
  — Wall-hung stainless steel sink for preparation of gastrointestinal contrast media solutions and for hand washing.
• The control area, including the operator's console, the radiologist's viewing desk, and the matrix camera, should have an area of at least 125 square feet and be rectangular.
• The computer, electronic rack cabinets, and transformer will need about 95 square feet.
  — The layout should allow for maintenance by providing ample access for service personnel to work behind the cabinets.

*Adapted from *Starting and Managing Your Radiology Imaging Center.* Winthrop Pharmaceuticals—Diagnostic Imaging Division.

—The computer room must be maintained at a constant 75 degrees Fahrenheit by an isolated air-conditioning system.

—Computer flooring is recommended.

• A dedicated darkroom nearby should be about 40 square feet.

• Lavatories for the patients who have CT studies must be conveniently located.

MRI Suite Layout

• The total area for the MRI system should be rectangular, with a floor space of about 2,500 square feet. Ceiling height should be at least 14 feet and be free of ferrous material.

—Access to all components for servicing is crucial.

—To allow for future expansion and upgrades, design the system on a 5-gauge field-strength limit with a magnet size of 2 tesla.

—Place system on ground floor with no basement so that one dimension of the magnetic field is directed in the earth.

—Design foundation to accept stress tolerances of 490,000 N/M2.

—Heat dissipation requirements will be approximately 400,000 BTUs per hour.

• The imaging room should be about 40 feet by 25 feet.

• The control room should be about 125 square feet in area.

Appendix C

Selected Accessibility Guidelines from the
U.S. Architectural and Transportation
Barriers Compliance Board

Suite 1000
1331 F Street, N.W.
Washington, D.C. 20004-1111
202/272-5434 (Voice)
202/272-5449 (TDD)

August 1992

Dimensions of Adult-Sized Wheelchairs

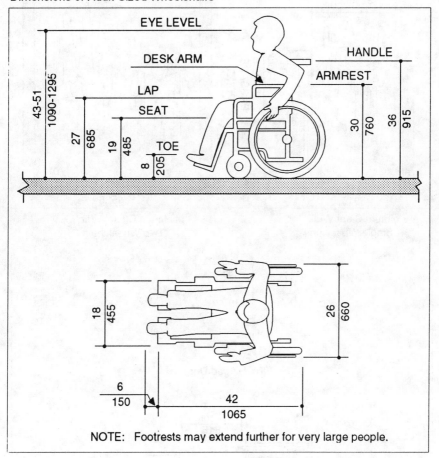

NOTE: Footrests may extend further for very large people.

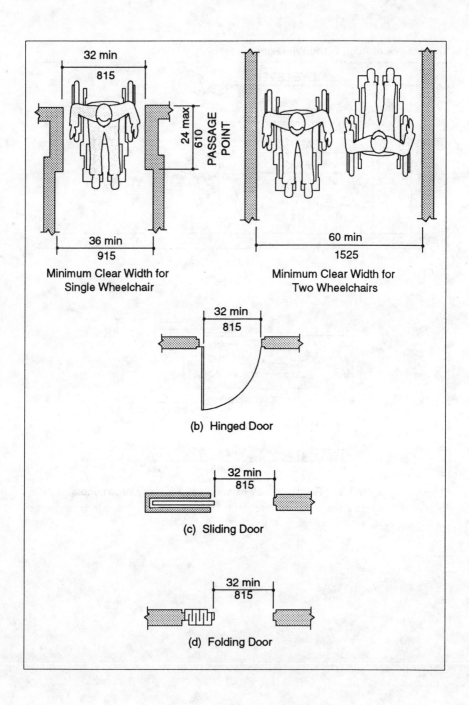

32 min
815

24 max
610

PASSAGE POINT

36 min
915

Minimum Clear Width for Single Wheelchair

60 min
1525

Minimum Clear Width for Two Wheelchairs

32 min
815

(b) Hinged Door

32 min
815

(c) Sliding Door

32 min
815

(d) Folding Door

Space Allowances and Reach Ranges

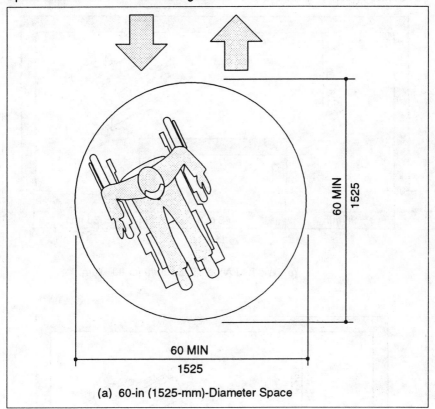

(a) 60-in (1525-mm)-Diameter Space

Accessible Routes and Ground and Floor Surfaces

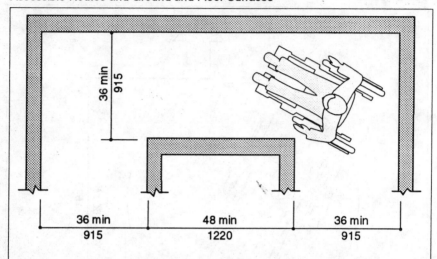

36 min
915

36 min
915

48 min
1220

36 min
915

(a) Width of Accessible Route for 90° Turn

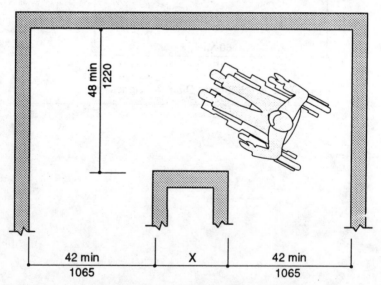

48 min
1220

42 min
1065

X

42 min
1065

NOTE: Dimensions shown apply when *x* < 48 in (1220 mm).

(b) Width of Accessible Route for Turns around an Obstruction

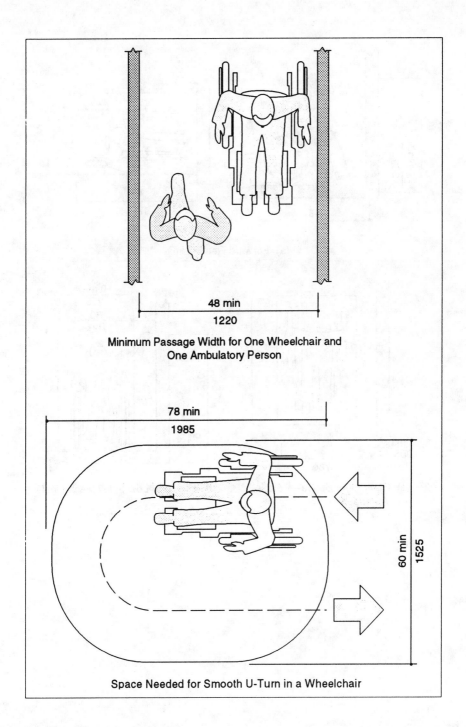

48 min
1220

Minimum Passage Width for One Wheelchair and
One Ambulatory Person

78 min
1985

60 min
1525

Space Needed for Smooth U-Turn in a Wheelchair

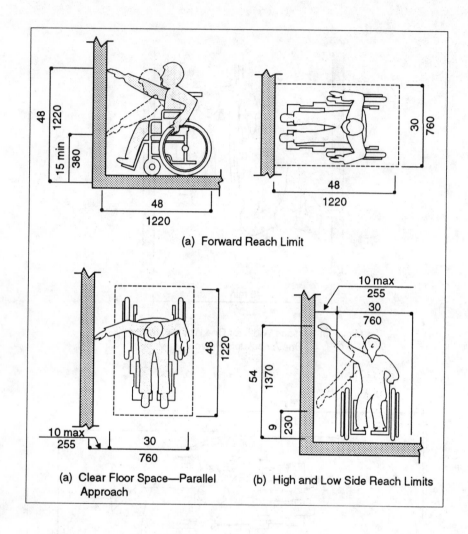

(a) Forward Reach Limit

(a) Clear Floor Space—Parallel
      Approach

(b) High and Low Side Reach Limits

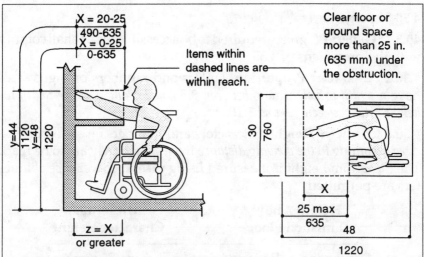

NOTE: x = Reach distance. y = Maximum hieght. z = Clear knee space. z is the clear space below the obstruction which shall be at least as deep as the reach distance, x.

(b) Maximum Forward Reach over an Obstruction

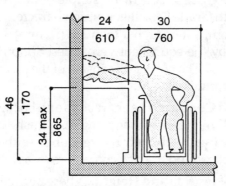

(c) Maximum Side Reach over Obstruction

Side Reach

4.30 Signage.

40.3.1* General. Signage required to be accessible by 4.1 shall comply with the provisions of 4.30.

4.30.2* Character Proportion. Letters and numbers on signs shall have a *width-to-height ratio between 3:5 and 1:1 and a stroke-width-to-height ratio between 1:5 and 1:10.*

4.30.3 Character Height. Characters and numbers on signs shall be *sized according to the viewing distance* from which they are to be read. The minimum height is measured using case X. Lower case characters are permitted.

Height Above Finished Floor	Minimum Character Height
Suspended or Projected Overhead in compliance with 4.4.2	*3 in.* (75 mm) minimum

4.30.4* Raised and Brailled Characters and Pictorial Symbol Signs (Pictograms). Leters and numerals shall be raised 1/32 in (0.8 mm) minimum, upper case, sans serif or simple serif type and shall be accompanied with Grade 2 Braille. Raised characters shall be at least 5/8 in (16 mm) high, but no higher than *2 in* (50 mm). Pictograms shall be accompanied by the equivalent verbal description placed directly below the pictogram. The border dimension of the pictogram shall be 6 in (152 mm) minimum in height.

4.30.5* Finish and Contrast. The characters and background of signs shall be eggshell, matte, or other nonglare finish. Characters and symbols shall contrast with their background—either light characters on a dark background or dark characters on a light background.

4.30.6 Mounting Location and Height. Where permanent identification is provided for rooms and spaces, signs shall be installed on the wall adjacent to the latch side of the door. Where there is no wall space to the latch side of the door, including at double leaf doors, signs shall be placed on the nearest adjacent wall. *Mounting height shall be 60 in* (1525 mm) above the finish floor to the centerline of the sign. Mounting location for such signage shall be so that a person may approach within 3 in (76 mm) of signage without encountering protruding objects or standing within the swing of a door.

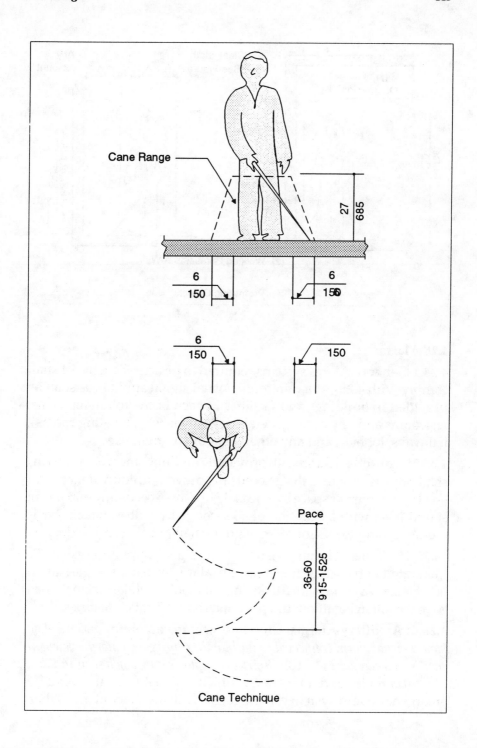

Cane Range

27
685

6
150

6
150

6
150

150

Pace

36-60
915-1525

Cane Technique

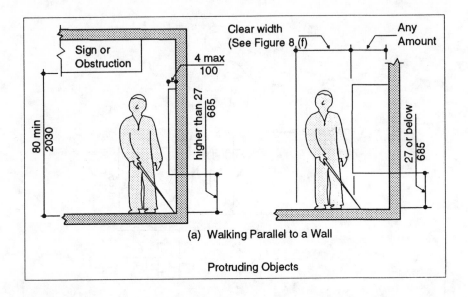

Sign or Obstruction

Clear width (See Figure 8 (f))

Any Amount

4 max
100

80 min
2030

higher than 27
685

27 or below
685

(a) Walking Parallel to a Wall

Protruding Objects

4.28 Alarms

4.28.1 General. Alarm systems required to be accessible by 4.1 shall comply with 4.28. At a minimum, visual signal appliances shall be provided in buildings and facilities in each of the following areas: restrooms and any other general usage areas (e.g., meeting rooms), hallways, lobbies, and any other area for common use.

4.28.2* Audible Alarms. If provided, audible emergency alarms shall produce a sound that exceeds the prevailing equivalent sound level in the room or space by at least 15 dbA or exceeds any maximum sound level with a duration of 60 seconds by 5 dbA, whichever is louder. Sound levels for alarm signals shall not exceed 120 dbA.

4.28.3* Visual Alarms. Visual alarm signal appliances shall be integrated into the building or facility alarm system. If single station audible alarms are provided then single station visual alarm signals shall have the following minimum photometric and location features.

4.28.4* Auxiliary Alarms. Units and sleeping accommodations *shall have a visual alarm connected to the building emergency alarm system or shall have a standard 110-volt electrical receptacle into which such an alarm can be connected* and a means by which a signal from the building emergency alarm system can trigger such an auxiliary alarm. When visual alarms are in place the signal shall be visible in all areas of the unit or room. Instructions for use of the auxiliary alarm or receptacle shall be provided.

1. *The lamp shall be a xenon strobe type or equivalent.*
2. The color shall be clear or nominal white (i.e., unfiltered or clear filtered white light).
3. *The maximum pulse duration shall be two-tenths of one second (0.2 sec) with a maximum duty cycle of 40 percent.* The pulse duration is defined as the time interval between initial and final points of 10 percent of maximum signal.
4. *The intensity* shall be a minimum of *75 candela.*
5. The flash rate shall be a minimum of 1 Hz and a maximum of 3 Hz.
6. *The appliance shall be placed 80 in (2030 mm) above the highest floor level within the space or 6 in (152 mm) below the ceiling,* whichever is lower.
7. In general, *no place in any room or space required to have a visual signal appliance shall be more than 50 ft (15 m) from the signal* (in the horizontal plane). In large rooms and spaces exceeding 100 ft (30 m) across, without obstructions 6 ft (2 m) above the finish floor, such as auditoriums, devices may be placed around the perimeter, spaced a maximum 100 ft (30 m) apart, in lieu of suspending appliances from the ceiling.
8. *No place in common corridors or hallways in which visual alarm signalling appliances are required shall be more than 50 ft (15 m) from the signal.*

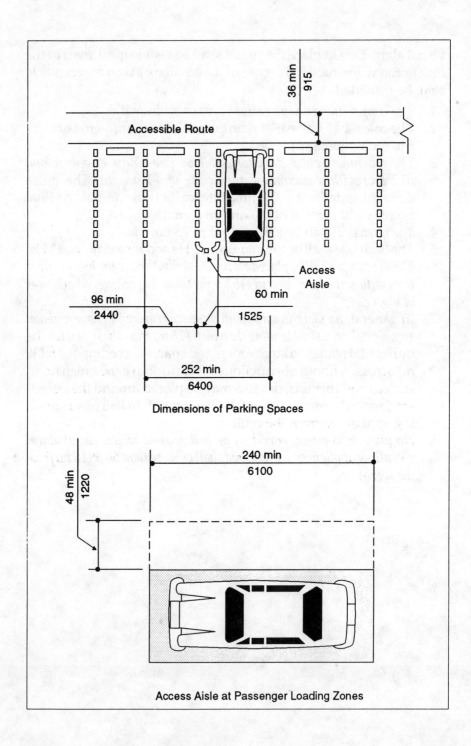

Accessible Route

Access
Aisle

36 min
915

96 min
2440

60 min
1525

252 min
6400

Dimensions of Parking Spaces

240 min
6100

48 min
1220

Access Aisle at Passenger Loading Zones

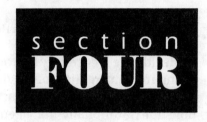

section
FOUR

MANAGING

4.1 SERVICE LINE MANAGEMENT

4.2 THE NEW MANAGER

4.3 TOTAL QUALITY MANAGEMENT

4.4 RADIOLOGY BENCHMARKING

4.5 COST CONTAINMENT

4.6 LICENSURE OF RADIOLOGIC PROFESSIONALS

4.7 JOINT VENTURES

4.8 THE JOINT COMMISSION ON ACCREDITATION
OF HEALTHCARE ORGANIZATIONS

4.9 RISK MANAGEMENT AND LIABILITY PREVENTION

4.10 BASIC HEALTHCARE FINANCIAL MANAGEMENT

4.11 QUALITY–ASSESSMENT AND IMPROVEMENT

4.1   SERVICE LINE MANAGEMENT

Healthcare is currently borrowing from industry concepts related to the implementation of service line management. This management concept suggests innovations that have far-reaching implications for traditionally managed medical centers. Service line management fits the hospital environment well. The focus is on defining who and what we are as a business (imaging in this case) and having a management person assigned to coordinate the needs of the service in a manner that allows for quicker, more responsive, and thus better imaging products.

The service line concept has evolved from the examples set in big business in this country. Service line thinking emerges from the realization that healthcare produces many different services which need specialized market analysis, sales strategies, and unique distribution plans. Service line management benefits the organization in a number of ways:

- It forces accountability for operations and results into the energies of one manager.
- It encourages coordination of services with various other activities in the organization.
- It promotes market analysis and the identification of specific target groups as potential customers.
- It links together strategic planning, operations, and program evaluation.

Who Is the Service Line Manager?

Lindsey Bradley, CEO of Mother Francis Regional Medical Center in Tyler, Texas, suggests that service line managers may have different profiles. Bradley's experiences suggest that a manager with a technical orientation demonstrates a greater potential for success in leading the activities associated with new major service lines such as oncology, cardiology, neurosciences, surgery, renal/nephrology, and emergency medicine. Experience as a generalist requires that an individual learn the technical nuances of a service.

The real challenge is to utilize the best characteristics of the manager; sometimes that's the manager with the technical orientation who learns general management principles. Or, a generalist in administration is selected that displays the potential to learn the specifics of a technical area.

Focus on Service

Traditional hospital organizational charts allow too many issues to get caught in the cracks of departmental lines. The service line function allows administration to respond to current issues in patient care without the burden of endless committee structure and reporting protocols. It promotes a spirit of "let's fix it," and physicians like service line management because it is efficient! A doctor doesn't have to talk to four different department heads to resolve an issue. With service line, reaction to the issue is facilitated by the person charged to get the necessary changes accomplished. Service line management improves the quality of hospital care. It gets the hospital's organization closer to the patient and to the physician.

Service Line Organization

A service line orientation requires a structural reconfiguration of the organizational chart. Functional directors with classic hospital-type responsibilities are replaced with service line people who report directly to the CEO. These individuals become responsible for the full menu of hospital care that is rendered to a specific consumer population. There is some flattening of the administrative structure of senior management. Fewer assistant administrators are required with the service line model. A table of organization similar to that described here could be found in institutions adopting the product line approach. The number of prospective service lines will differ according to the specific programs the hospital wishes to maintain.

Imaging as a Service Line

So, who are these new service line professionals? They are individuals who are skilled in marketing and planning, financial analysis, negotiation, and problem solving. Service line managers are entrepreneurial and have a clear idea about future directions. They have clinical experience and maintain good medical staff relations. The ability to relate to medical staff concerns is of paramount importance. It is traditional for strong medical staff involvement in decision making to exist in successful hospitals.

Managing imaging has been a service line activity in most healthcare institutions for quite some time. It is not surprising then, that service line managers in institutions are rising from the ranks of radiology. Radiology managers already possess the management skills required of service line managers. These skills are easily transferable and expandable to encompass other hospital activities.

4.2   THE NEW MANAGER

The clinician-to-manager transition is an often found phenomenon in the field of radiology management. When a clinician wants to advance his career, stepping up into a management position is just about the only option available in the narrow supervisory hierarchy that exists in the imaging industry today. Being a good clinician, however, does not ensure that those technical skills will translate into successful management techniques. Consider some of these questions when evaluating whether to make that move into full-time management.

1) Do You Really Want to Do the Work of a Manager?

If you think your boss has an easy job, well take a closer look. Spend time observing the boss; consider whether you really want to do those daily activities of supervision. Don't let your desire to advance cloud your expectations about job satisfaction. You may be aspiring to a job status that ends up being undesirable. There are many examples of clinicians trapped in the role of manager, leaving them ineffective supervisors and unrewarded on the job. Weigh the financial rewards of leaving the clinical ranks very carefully. Often a clinician can make more money than his supervisor through overtime, differentials, bonuses, and other compensation.

2) Is There Management Training Available to Prepare You for a Promotion?

Hopefully the organization you are in recognizes the importance of career development. Management or supervisory development opportunities can be as simple as tuition reimbursement or as detailed as counseling services for developing individual career plans. Organizations choosing to promote aspects of career development for employees will have training plans in effect that attend to key elements of career development to include some of the following:

- Career counseling.
- Planned job progression.
- Career information.
- Management and supervisory development.
- Training.
- Special plans (i.e., outplacement, preretirement counseling, minority interests).

3) How Can You Ensure Your Success as a New Supervisor?

Look for opportunities to ease into management tasks by seeking out managerial experiences. Volunteer to organize a certain aspect of department operations such as overseeing time cards, film badge monitoring, or special projects. Over time, an accumulation of these experiences places you in a logical position to move up when a supervisory opening occurs.

Brush up on "people skills." New managers find that dealing with subordinates brings unanticipated challenges. Clinicians who become managers are vulnerable to the tendency to revert to old habits like performing comfortable clinical tasks rather than delegating them. Those difficult tasks of management that require great interpersonal skills such as coaching and motivating workers need to be learned. Seek out a mentor that you consider to be a good manager. The experienced manager can serve as a role model and advisor.

Identifying Your Management Style

A great manager understands that management style needs to conform to the values and motives of employees as well as the mission and goals of the organization. Different circumstances dictate different management styles. A talented manager will blend different management styles to best suit the occasion.

Some Leading Management Styles

Coach managers help employees develop by identifying strengths and weaknesses. Coach managers let employees set their own goals and assign problem solving.

Democratic managers build employee consensus. These managers are very interested in hearing employee ideas and using their input to improve the work environment.

Authoritative managers make clear and concise directives and explain the reasons for the directions.

Coercive managers use threats and discipline to get employees in line. This style is ineffective in most situations.

Pacesetting managers are example oriented. They usually do not delegate authority and get along well as long as employees are highly motivated. This technique of leading by example is more effective when blended with another management style.

Habits of Very Effective Managers

The major responsibility of a manager today is the efficient use of human resources. Managers that are successful work at it constantly. Most successful managers have habits in common that characterize them as successful people. They are:

- **Independence.** Great managers are willing to accept responsibility for developing solutions and can do so alone.
- **Listening Skills.** Most people do not listen with the intent to understand; they listen with the intent to reply. Effective managers focus on what is being said and really think about it before responding.
- **Self-Discipline.** Successful managers understand that you cannot control anything until you control yourself. They understand that they must perform even unpleasant tasks with the same level of professionalism.

- **Understanding**. Life and business are about people. Crucial to success is the ability to recognize what makes people act as they do and to develop relationships.
- **Teamwork**. The most effective managers recognize that the balance derived from working with others yields far greater results than is possible alone.
- **Negotiation Skills**. The ability to commit to establishing a win-win situation is a strong skill to learn and practice consistently.
- **Creativity**. Developing the habit of looking at things differently and striving to improve situations is what makes the process of work fun.

Strategies for Being a Successful New Manager

Taking charge requires talent, thought, and strategy. Capitalize on opportunities and strategies that will help your chances of success at being in charge and staying in charge!

- Be aggressive about your arrival in a new organization. Announcements in in-house publications and local newspapers need to tell people who you are. Visit other department heads, medical staff, and senior management. Find out how your new place of employment functions.
- Take on some issues that yield immediate results. Employees who recognize their new leader as an advocate will get in line to be supportive. Use a "new broom sweeps clean" attitude to identify some long-standing problems and tackle those issues for positive results.
- Create a management style through your own actions. For example, start the work day at the same time you expect your subordinates to begin. Model the behavior you expect from others.
- Raise performance expectations in ways that communicate to employees that there is a new vision in management. Build a new management team that understands and buys into the results you want to achieve.

4.3   TOTAL QUALITY MANAGEMENT

Quality

Quality is and is expected to remain one of the dominant issues of the 1990s. The focus on quality rests on the idea that in the healthcare industry in particular we can do a much better job of meeting customer needs. The healthcare industry, like all industries in this society, has focused its attention on the internal workings of the organization rather than on the customer and the organization's future. This production-oriented emphasis has been a detriment to the way the healthcare industry is perceived at large. In a production-oriented climate, the debate and argument becomes one of relationships and delegation. When orientation switches to quality, the perspective on getting the work done moves towards working together and meeting customer needs. The work done by W. Edwards Deming, J.P. Juran, and Phillip Crosby (among others) centers on two main ideas that have become the foundation of total quality management theory. The first is **conformance to customer expectations**. An organization should do what the customer expects. Customers have specific requirements for products or services, and the organization must center on meeting those customer expectations. What this means is not providing less or more but providing exactly what the customer wants. The second basic idea of total quality management is **continuous improvement**. It is the emerging consensus that successful quality efforts are based on continuous improvement, that is, the ideology that things can always get better. Continuous improvement focuses on meeting customer expectations, anticipating future needs, and simplifying operations to accomplish what is needed more effectively. See figure 4.1 for one physician's view of quality in healthcare.

Figure 4.1   10

---

1.   *In the hassle-free hospital, everyone treats everyone else as a customer.* For example, physicians treat ward clerks with respect and communicate with

them routinely, not just when there are problems. Conversely, lab clerks treat the emergency physicians as customers, making the extra effort to efficiently send lab techs and lab results to the emergency department (ED).

A customer focus starts with a simple premise: All health care team members know that they are in the hospital to serve others, just as they depend on others to do their job right.

A physician should always identify the patient as the first customer. But a physician's customers also include the nurse, who helps take care of the patient, and those who help them (ward clerk, tray aide, housekeeper).

2. *Radiology and lab reports get onto the chart in a timely manner.*
It is vital for attending and referral physicians to be able to obtain important radiology and lab data in a timely manner, particularly for same-day surgery patients. But there are many potential rate-limiting steps in this process. The order has to be taken off the chart, transmitted, and received; the test has to be performed; then the result obtained, transmitted, and entered on the chart. At some hospitals, this may involve five, 10, or 20 steps and take hours or days. Finding the 20 percent of the steps that cause 80 percent of the delays will help create the hassle-free hospital.

3. *The person who answers the phone when you respond to a page knows why you were paged.* Few situations are more exasperating to a physician than to be paged to a hospital floor and, when responding, no one seems to know the purpose for the page.

4. *Nurses learn the names of patients' families and visitors.* Hassle-free hospitals encourage staff members to identify family members and visitors. This comforts them as well as the patient. Of course this means there are enough nurses around on a regular basis to learn the family members' names.

5. *Nurses know where their patients are at all times.* When a nurse doesn't know where a patient is, it isn't always due to inattention. Nurses can easily lose track of patients in understaffed units. Understaffing occurs partly as a result of unnecessary non-patient care tasks being performed by nurses.
In a hassle-free hospital, when a nurse is asked where a patient is, the nurse knows without having to consult four different clipboards.

6. *Both radiology and the operating room allow time for work-ins.* Radiology departments and operating rooms need to make time, rooms, and personnel available for emergency work-ins. A hassle-free hospital realizes that patients don't get sick by appointment.

7. *Chairmen of clinical departments make decisions.* At medical executive committee meetings, chairmen make decisions as representatives of their departments. They don't have to take every decision back to their department to ask every physician's opinion, resulting in further delay.

8. *Clinical personnel from different disciplines sit down together.* For example, surgeons, operating room nurses and administrators meet monthly on an operating room committee to solve problems.

9. *Meetings have agendas, and they start and end on time,* increasing the likelihood of future attendance.

10. *Patients receive a daily schedule of what's going to happen to them.* This may sound like a fantasy, but it can happen. A natural extension of the creation of critical pathways would be for a patient to receive a schedule in the morning of the tests and procedures to be done that day, as well as a list of best times for visitors. Now that's exceeding your customer's expectations.

Adapted from: Musfeldt, C. The Last Word: 10 Attributes of a hassle-free hospital. *Hospitals.* August 20, 1992. p. 76.

What Is Total Quality Management?

Total quality management is considered to be the most important and exciting change in the way that American healthcare institutions are providing care. The healthcare delivery system is being impacted by a fundamental quality improvement philosophy which is comprehensive, practical in approach, and realistic in expectations. Total quality management views work as a dynamic process, and whether the issues are clinical or managerial, it recognizes that people need to work together in an effective manner to get things accomplished. Total quality management helps people see the big picture so that the immediacy of their own tasks and roles fit into the work of others. Total quality management is a new paradigm of cooperation and team spirit.

The Quality Vision

Total quality management is a top-down process. Senior management must shape and communicate this unified vision of quality and serve as coaches to all remaining levels of management engaged in the quality improvement process. Without the visible support of top hospital leadership, the program will lose momentum and flounder from loss of direction.

Total quality management is a value-driven process. The central value of all quality improvement activities is *customer satisfaction*. This customer satisfaction value is expanded to include patients, physicians, insurers, and organizations that offer preferred provider opportunities. All of these "customers" guide the principles of continuous improvement. The concept of continuous improvement dictates that there is always the potential to do better. It becomes everyone's responsibility to constantly seek better ways to meet customer needs.

Benchmarking drives the TQM process*

Thousands of firms are now benchmarking. Why?

First, benchmarking accelerates the rate of improvement. When you were born, if you had had to reinvent reading and writing, it

---

* Adapted from: O'Dell, C. Building on received wisdom. *Healthcare Forum Journal*. 36(1): 17-8, 1993.

would have taken a long time. Fortunately, it already had been done. The whole course of human history is about building on received wisdom. Accelerating the rate of change in an organization includes building on the wisdom of others and being open to adopting innovations from elsewhere.

Second, benchmarking can help you identify breakthroughs. If you understand your own process and you find others who do it much better, you may be able to adopt their breakthrough. In fact, some of the most dramatic improvements in cost and cycle time reduction come from finding out you don't even *need* to do a process at all; someone else has discovered a way to eliminate it.

Third, people benchmark to improve customer satisfaction. Probably the largest paradigm shift in the quality movement during the last five years has been a change from an internal focus on improvement-understand your process and make it better-to looking outward and saying, "It doesn't matter whether *we* like the process; what does the *customer* say?"

Finally, benchmarking helps you gain consensus. Instead of relying on a personal opinion about who is better and what is a superior way to do things, there are real external data and knowledge about how others do it. See Figure 4.2 for benchmarking steps.

Figure 4.2 Four Steps to Successful Benchmarking

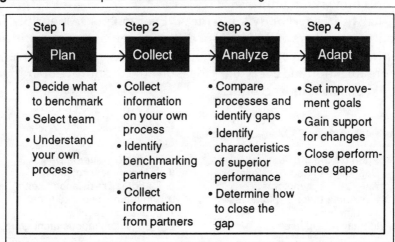

Step 1	Step 2	Step 3	Step 4
Plan	**Collect**	**Analyze**	**Adapt**
• Decide what to benchmark	• Collect information on your own process	• Compare processes and identify gaps	• Set improvement goals
• Select team	• Identify benchmarking partners	• Identify characteristics of superior performance	• Gain support for changes
• Understand your own process	• Collect information from partners	• Determine how to close the gap	• Close performance gaps

Improving the Process

The fundamental mechanics of process improvement are modeled after the scientific method. This adapted method consists of 12 problem-solving steps which guide the quality improvement process. (See Figure 4.3) Critical activities such as patient registration, transportation, file jacket management, and procedure turnaround are best analyzed and improved when they're viewed as parts of a chain in an overall system. All parts of the delivery system must work together on the behalf of the customer.

Typically, a quality improvement group is organized to identify and prioritize key issues to work on. When issues involve interdepartmental concerns, the group is expanded to accommodate the responsible managers. (See Figure 4.4) W. Edwards Deming is notably the top quality expert in the country today. His 14 points of total quality management can serve as a philosophical framework for your quality improvement programming. (See Figure 4.5) Appendix A lists resources available to those who wish to study TQM in further detail.

Principles for a Sound Quality Effort

Quality can always get better. Never be satisfied with the way things are done or your ability to serve customers. We can always get better at what we do. In successful organizations, management focuses on ways to improve.

Quality is everybody's business. Everyone is responsible for quality—members of the board of directors, senior managers, every employee. Discussions about quality should occur at every level of the organization and everyone's ideas on how to improve operations should be taken into account.

Figure 4.3 Twelve Problem-Solving Steps

1.	Prioritize the problem.	7.	Consider alternatives.
2.	Define the project and team.	8.	Design new solutions.
3.	Analyze the symptoms.	9.	Address resistance to change.
4.	Formulate theories of causes.	10.	Implement new solutions.
5.	Test theories.	11.	Evaluate results.
6.	Identify root causes.	12.	Begin continuous monitoring.

Figure 4.4 Total Quality Management

Corrective Maintenance Program Project

PROBLEM

The current process for the repair and continued preventive maintenance of capital equipment is fragmented and expensive. The result is a cost excessive system of maintenance and repair.

RECOMMENDED TASK FORCE PARTICIPANTS
- Vice President Professional Services
- Director of Imaging Services
- Director of Materials Management
- Director of Biomedical Engineering (Task Force Leader)
- Director of Critical Care Nursing
- Director of Surgical Services
- Director of Respiratory Care
- Director of Medical Laboratories

GOAL

To develop a comprehensive maintenance program for all hospital equipment which is cost efficient and responsive to the requirements of all users.

OBJECTIVES
- Increase uptime of medical equipment.
- Faster response time of service engineers.
- Improved coordination and control of equipment repair records.
- Decreased costs of equipment repair.
- Increased satisfaction of staff.

BARRIERS
- Cooperation of individual department managers in a system of centralization and standardization.
- Resistance of department managers to give up control of repair issues within their area of responsibility.
- Availability of personnel to manage a hospital-wide corrective maintenance program.

TIME FRAME

Meetings will be held biweekly. A recommendation to administration will be made at the end of 60 days.

New ideas are everywhere. Every idea is a possible opportunity for quality improvement. Organizations that operate under total quality management principles encourage managers to listen to employees.

Quality efforts should be consistently implemented. Follow-through on the implementation of quality efforts is monitored. Quality management needs to be uniformly administered. That is, quality improvement groups operate in the same manner in every department.

Figure 4.5 The 14 Points of W. Edwards Deming

1. Create constancy of purpose for the improvement of product and service.
2. Adopt the new philosophy.
3. Cease dependence on mass inspection.
4. End the practice of awarding business on price tag alone.
5. Improve constantly and forever the system of production and service.
6. Institute training and retraining.
7. Institute leadership.
8. Drive out fear.
9. Break down barriers between staff areas.
10. Eliminate slogans, exhortations, and targets for the workforce.
11. Eliminate numerical quotas.
12. Remove barriers to pride in workmanship.
13. Institute a vigorous program of education and retraining.
14. Take action to accomplish the transformation.

Quality improvement depends upon collaboration. Collaboration and work across departmental lines is a key to sound quality efforts. Successful quality management efforts have demonstrated that quality improvement can occur among divisions and departments rather than within the individual departments or divisions themselves.

Quality management requires patience. A total quality management program sees results with sustained hard work over long periods of time. Total quality management programs have a focus on consistent long-term improvement rather than a quick fix mentality.

Quality management needs dependable data. An organization committed to total quality management must identify what is important to accomplish to meet customer needs and to continuously improve for the future. Data must be collected on important indicators of quality.

Quality management requires training. Quality doesn't simply happen; it depends upon training in the methods and the procedures of the quality management. Skills that employees will need in order to effectively direct quality efforts include coordination skills, facilitation skills (see facilitator selection critiria figure 4.6), data management abilities, and basic human relations development. Even though the training budgets in quality based organizations will significantly increase, the total cost of doing business as a result of quality improvement interventions will come down.

Quality management improves management reporting. Traditional management systems change in order to accommodate the

Figure 4.6 Facilitator Selection Criteria

1. People from different levels within the organization. 2. People who have credibility. 3. People with a track record of success. 4. People who are known to be team players and have leadership ability. 5. People with good communication skills. 6. People who volunteered.

tenets of total quality management. New monitoring tools are generated that form the basis for management discussions that are focused on results, improved satisfaction, and the continuously improved processes. Better management reporting information throughout an organization makes management more effective.

Based on the aforementioned principles for a sound quality effort, a self-assessment survey for any organization can be developed to determine where that organization is in undertaking a quality effort. The self-assessment tool included here is adapted from the Westrend Group, Denver, Colorado. Another self-evalution tool is described in Appendix B.

Quality Self-Assessment Survey

	Yes	No	In Progress

Data management:
1. We have identified essential elements to monitor a quality effort.
2. We have assembled the data to monitor our quality effort.
3. We have begun to eliminate redundant or duplicative information.
4. We have identified additional information we need to focus on to monitor quality.
5. We have identified information we can stop collecting because it is not central to our success in serving customers.

Training:
1. The board has been exposed to the ideas of quality.
2. Senior staff and managers have attended quality training programs.
3. Staff throughout the organization regularly participates in quality training programs.
4. Our investment in human resources and training is going up each year.

Management/monitoring systems:
1. We regularly use quality charts in management meetings.
2. We regularly assemble teams from different departments to make improvements in what we do and how we do it.

Measuring Success

Measuring the success of total quality management is the result of many small changes that when accumulated add up to major improvements. The process teaches techniques that empower people to identify and deal with key systemic weaknesses. Quality improvement focuses intellectual energy on the task of eliminating underlying inefficiencies in the workplace. There is a definite connection between quality improvement and operational efficiency; the connection is employees solving problems in a planned systematic manner.

Appendix A—Total Quality Management

Sources of Additional Information

Books:

Teaching the Elephant to Dance: Empowering Change in Your Organization by James A. Belasco. Crown Publishers, Inc., New York, New York, 1990.

The Service Edge: A Hundred and One Companies That Profit from Customer Care by Ron Zemke with Dick Schraff and a foreword by Tom Peters. A Plume Book, New York, New York, 1989.

The Service Advantage: How to Identify and Fulfill Customer Needs by Carl Albrecht and Lawrence J. Bradford. Dow Jones-Irwin Publisher, Homewood, Illinois, 1990.

Implementing Total Quality Management: Competing in the 1990's by Joseph R. Jablonski with a foreword by Paul Hartman. Published by Technical Management Consortium, Inc., Albuquerque, New Mexico, 1990.

When America Does It Right: Case Studies in Service Quality by J. W. Spechler. Industrial Engineering and Management Press, Norcross, Georgia, 1991.

Out of the Crisis by W. Edwards Deming. Massachusetts Institute of Technology, Cambridge, Massachusetts, 1982.

Quality Process Management by Gabriela A. Paull. Prentice-Hall Company, Inc., Inglewood Cliffs, New Jersey, 1987.

Current Healthcare: New Strategies for Quality Improvement by Donald M. Berwick with A. Blanton Godfrey and Jane Roessner. Jossey-Bass Publishers, San Francisco, California, 1991.

Quality is Free: The Art of Making Quality Certain by Philip B. Crosby. New American Library, New York, New York, 1979.

Quality Without Tears: The Art of Hassle-Free Management by Philip B. Crosby. A Plumme Book, New York, New York, 1984.

Building a Chain of Customers: Linking Business Functions to Create the World Class Company by Richard J. Schonberger. The Free Press, New York, New York, 1990.

Delivering Quality Service: Balancing Customer Perceptions and Expectations by Valarie A. Zeithamel with A. Parasuraman and Leonard L. Berry. The Free Press, New York, New York, 1990.

Guide to Quality Control by Kaoru Ishikawa. Published by Quality Resources, White Plains, New York, 1982.

Let's Talk Quality: 96 Questions You Always Wanted to Ask Phil Crosby by Philip B. Crosby. McGraw-Hill Publishing Company, New York, New York, 1989.

Managing the Total Quality Transformation by Thomas H. Berry with a foreword by A. Blanton Godfrey, Chairman and CEO of The Juran Institute. McGraw-Hill Inc., New York, New York, 1990.

Other Sources of Information on Total Quality Management:

The AOP Report: The Newsletter for Quality and Participation. Association for Quality and Participation, 801-B West 8th St., Cincinnati, OH 45203.

Quality Connection: News from the National Demonstration Project on Quality Improvement in Healthcare. National Demonstration Project c/o Harvard Community Health Plan, 10 Brookline Place West, Brookline, MA 02146.

On "Q": The Official Newsletter of the American Society for Quality Control. ASQC, P. O. Box 3005, Milwaukee, WI 53201

QI/TQM: The Healthcare Executive's Guide to Quality Improvement Through Total Quality Management. A newsletter published by Warren B. Causey, American Health Consultants, P. O. Box 740056, Atlanta, GA 30374.

American Society for Quality Control, 310 W. Wisconsin Avenue, Suite 500, Milwaukee, WI 53203.

American Productivity and Quality Center, 123 N. Post Oak Lane, Houston, Texas 77024.

Association for Quality and Participation, 801 B. West 8th Street, Cincinnati, Ohio 45203.

Appendix B

*Where is Your Organization in Terms of Quality?**

Characteristics	That's us all the way	Some is true	We're not like that
1. Our services and/or products normally contain waivers, deviations, and other indications of not conforming to requirements.			

* From Jablonski, J.R. Implementing Total Quality Management in the 1990's. Technical Management Consortium, Inc. Albuquerque, N.M., 1991, p. 81.

2. We have a "fix it" oriented field service and/or dealer organization.

3. Our employees do not know what management wants from them concerning quality.

4. Management does not know what the price of nonconformance really is.

5. Management believes that quality is a problem caused by something other than management action.

5 Points   3 Points   1 Point

Point count condition		
21-25	Critical	Needs intensive care immediately.
16-20	Guarded	Needs life support system-hookup.
11-15	Resting	Needs medication and attention.
6-10	Healing	Needs regular checkup.
5	Whole	Needs Counseling

Appendix C

First Step in Initiating an Improvement Project

QUALITY IMPROVEMENT RECOMMENDATION

TO: Director, Quality Improvement

FROM: _____   DEPARTMENT: _____

DATE: _____   PHONE: _____

What is the problem or process that needs to be improved? _____

_____

_____

_____

Who will be impacted by creating this team? _____

_____

_____

_____

_____

How will we know if the problem is solved or the process improved?

_____

_____

_____

_____

_____

Who do you think should be represented on this proposed quality improvement team: _____

_____

_____

_____

_____

_____

_____

Appendix D

How to improve service between departments

We usually think of service as "customer relations." But people who must cooperate with each other on the job perform equally important "internal service."

Unfortunately, sometimes departments within an organization seem to be working against each other rather than in cooperation. They antagonize each other with delays or denials. Not only is this behavior annoying, it is inefficient and harms business.

Consultant Karl Albrecht has identified "Seven Sins" that internal service departments often commit. How many of these do you recognize?

1. **The Black Hole:** Things go in but nothing ever seems to come out. Requests for information, advice or special assistance seem to go unheeded. Departments operate as if they are autonomous and ignore other departments until management puts the heat on.

2. **The Bounce-Back** department enjoys rejecting requests on procedural grounds. "You didn't fill in line 24 of the standard Request Form, therefore we are returning your request without action." Instead of calling the department to get the missing information, they throw the request back in its face.

3. **The Edict:** A department enjoys making declarations of what they will or won't do in the future. "Effective today, we will no longer process budget requests without written notification signed by the supervisor." The message is, "This is how it's going to be; take it or leave it."

4. **The Gotcha** department polices others and gets carried away. They seem to take a sadistic pleasure in catching people in other departments making mistakes or violating rules. Internal audit, legal and affirmative action departments often fall into this role.

5. **No-ism** departments delight in exercising their veto power by telling others "No." Instead of a "can-do" attitude, they have a

Karl Albrecht, *Service Within*, Dow Jones-Irwin, 1818 Ridge Road, Homewood, IL 60430. As adapted by the Pryor Report Vol 9(1):9, 1993.

"No, you can't" attitude. Instead of saying "This can't be done," they should try to meet legitimate needs.

6. **The Papermill** department buries you in paperwork with special request forms. They won't discuss a problem over the phone and take immediate action. They want requests to be submitted in triplicate with fifteen signatures before they'll even decide to say yes or no.

7. **Turfism** is a department's jealous preoccupation with its responsibilities when common sense tells you compromise is necessary to get results. A "turfist" department may ignore a request from someone in another department, only to attack them when they decide to take action on their own.

Assess your organization's departments. What are their attitudes towards each other? Consult with the ones who have a reputation for "sinning." Affirm those who provide courteous, efficient internal service.

4.4 RADIOLOGY BENCHMARKING

Contributed by Alan Weinstein*

Measuring and improving performance may well become the keys to success for the hospital of the future; in many instances, they are being used to the advantage of the hospital of today. Premier Hospitals Alliance undertook its Radiology Best Practices Study at the request of member hospital chief operating officers, who sought to compare the performance of specific departments within their facilities to that achieved by the same departments at other hospitals, particularly in terms of quality and efficiency. While this approach is not new, the study's results do illustrate several easy, proven methods for improving hospital radiology departments and the services they provide.

The radiology benchmarking study used data collected by MECON Associates, San Ramon, Calif, for its MECON PEERx hospital-wide comparative data base. For the study, this data base provided infor-

---

* The article originally appeared in the Winter 1992 issue of *Decisions in Imaging Economics*. It is used with the permission of the author.

mation on six sections within radiology departments: diagnostic radiology (including special procedures), CT, MRI, nuclear medicine, ultrasound, and mammography.

Data collected for each of the six sections included:

- total procedures performed;
- employee hours worked and employee hours for which the department paid;
- percentage of section staff who were radiologic technologists and assistants;
- employee hours worked per procedure;
- labor expense per procedure;
- total expense per procedure;
- whether registered nurses and physicians were on the section's payroll;
- statistical characteristics, such as whether outpatient procedures accounted for more than 50% of total procedures and whether chest studies accounted for more than 40% of total procedures;
- organizational characteristics, such as whether staff provided training to others, transported patients, transcribed reports, or delivered and picked up film;
- operational characteristics, such as whether the section was open longer than 16 hours per day and whether it had automated order entry; and
- staffing characteristics, such as whether the department manager performed patient care during more than eight hours per week and whether scheduled staff hours were routinely cancelled, or whether staff were floated or given on-call responsibilities.

MECON collected data from 34 member hospitals and then provided a ranking of the five hospitals exhibiting the best performance in each radiology department section. Rankings were based upon hours worked per procedure and costs per procedure, with those hospitals reporting the fewest hours worked and lowest costs considered to have the best performance. In addition, MECON analyzed and reported the statistical, organizational, and operating characteristics of the five best performers.

Premier Hospitals Alliance subsequently identified the six hospitals showing the best overall performance by adding each hospital's section rankings and dividing the result by the number of sections in which the hospital was evaluated. The purpose of identifying the six best performers was to determine the factors responsible for their benchmark status.

To clarify those factors, graphs for overall best performers and best performers in each section were created. The first graph (Figure 4.7) arranged the hospitals according to size and demonstrated the performance of each according to labor costs and nonlabor costs as percentages of total costs per procedure. The second graph (Figure 4.8) plotted variances from average labor and nonlabor costs.

Dan Strauch, radiology administrator at Albert Einstein Medical Center, Philadelphia, says "The purpose of the study was not to point our hospitals with high costs, but to identify the best performers and then try to understand what factors in effect at those hospitals could help other hospitals improve their individual performances." He adds, "By sharing data among group members, we have learned more about the reasons for variances. Accounting for nonlabor costs, in particular, can skew results. Armed with that understanding, a hospital can investigate further to find the root causes of performance that may be out of line with the rest of the group."

Mark Goodhart, director of hospital relations for Premier Hospitals Alliance, says, "We look at the relative importance of labor costs versus nonlabor costs. If a hospital's total costs are too high, then the solution may not be labor-related. Shaving 15 minutes of labor off of a particular procedure may be insignificant and, in fact, counterproductive compared to working on nonlabor factors such as supplies or service agreements."

To make the comparative data more useful, Premier Hospitals Alliance conducted a second survey to identify variances in data reporting. With respect to nonlabor costs, the survey asked participating hospitals if they included depreciation, lease/rental costs, and service contracts. In addition, the survey asked if hospitals had assigned the cost of administrative personnel to the diagnostic radiology category or spread the cost over all six sections. Those factors made a significant difference in the results for several hospitals, particularly the extreme outliers.

The lesson learned is that looking at the performance of one section, such as diagnostic radiology, will not provide a complete

Figure 4.7 Roll-up–Labor and Nonlabor Cost. MECON PEERx data for costs at Premier Hospitals. Hospitals noted by number are the six best performers.

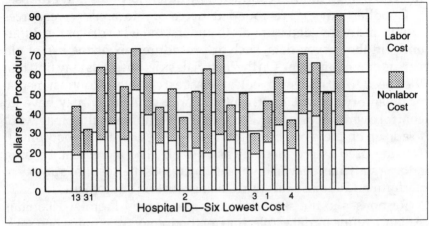

Figure 4.8 Roll-up–Variance Plot. Variances from average labor and nonlabor costs. Hospitals noted by number are the six best performers.

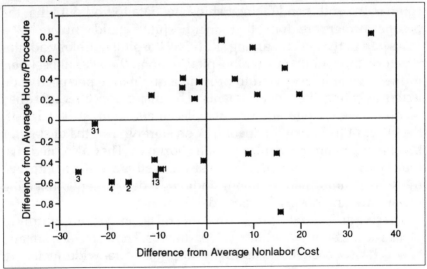

picture of how well a hospital is doing, according to George A. Wietmarschen, assistant vice president for imaging services at Jewish Hospital, Inc., Cincinnati. It is more important to look at the constellation of departments and know how the data for that constellation color the overall performance picture. This conclusion echoes those of similar studies conducted by other hospitals and groups.

Goodhart says, "We found it necessary to analyze resources within and across departments to understand what drives the differences in the survey data, such as procedure mix or the use of old versus new equipment. On the materials side, hospitals may find that they need to take a closer look at dosages, catheters, contrast media, or inventory control. On the other hand, while they may have no control over the costs of existing capital equipment, they may want to add an employee or cross-train staff to ensure that the equipment is being used as productively as possible. The incremental cost of adding staff may be worthwhile if it increases the hospital's ability to perform additional procedures using existing equipment."

Responses to the second survey also helped Premier Hospitals Alliance refine its data collection methodology. Wietmarschen says, "Our goal is to find sample data that will give all the hospitals the information that they need to become better. We have to start somewhere, looking critically at the data to make sure that they are comparable and then looking behind the data to find out what the best performers are doing that other hospitals could emulate."

As part of the benchmarking study, six hospital radiology administrators, three of them from hospitals among the overall best performers, were interviewed to provide a qualitative perspective on issues affecting their departments. The major concerns that they identified were capital equipment replacement, contrast media costs, the effect of a changing patient mix on staffing, lengths of stay for inpatients, reimbursement, and staff shortages. They also cited customer service and image quality issues, as well as a desire to improve the flow of information among radiology departments, referring physicians, and hospital finance departments.

The six administrators noted that several techniques are worthy of investigation by other radiology departments. These strategies, many of which have been found useful by hospitals nationwide, included:

- reducing nonionic contrast media costs by decreasing the standard dose from 150 cc to 100 cc, with larger doses ordered by radiologists as needed. During a three-week trial at one hospital, costs dropped by one-third.

- coordinating inpatient and outpatient flows. Several hospitals fill open slots with inpatients, and one schedules CT outpatients on the hour and begins to prep the next inpatient at the midpoint of the preceding patient's examination.
- cross-training staff to reduce the cost of keeping staff on call and on standby to meet unexpected demands. State licensure requirements and local labor markets can influence a hospital's ability to cross-train, however.
- using radiology assistants. Several member hospitals use assistants to handle clerical duties, run film, and escort patients as needed.
- hiring a patient advocate to improve communication between the technical staff and patients and to enhance patient satisfaction.
- using automated dictation, home computer terminals for radiologists, private couriers, and fax networks to access and deliver reports.
- developing an in-house radiology network, either by standardizing and linking SPECT units and sending images to a three-dimensional imaging station or by linking laser camera/processors to produce films from a variety of modalities.
- boosting productivity in particular modalities. One recommendation was to add a second console to an MRI unit to keep it in operation during the long processing time required for MRI angiography studies. A suggestion to speed CT studies was to use a pressure injector to administer contrast media and then to divide duties among an assistant, two technicians, and a physician.

The Radiology Best Practices Study represents a starting point for Premier Hospitals Alliance members in their radiology benchmarking efforts. Goodhart says, "This is an iterative process. We plan to conduct these studies on an ongoing basis to help our members improve their operations continuously."

4.5 COST CONTAINMENT

In today's hospital or free-standing imaging center, administrators find more and more that their attentions are focused on a daily basis towards competition and consumerism. The highly competitive nature of modern imaging poses the challenges of realizing optimum return on investment while keeping costs to a minimum.

Many hospitals are finding themselves in dire financial straits. Across the board financially distressed hospitals report similar difficulties: a large medicare population, a higher than average length of stay, aging medical staffs, technological obsolescence, and difficulty in recruiting and retaining professional staff. A reversal of fortune for these financial ills requires aggressive and immediate actions.

Financial Repositioning

When you hear your hospital administration saying it's "turnaround time," watch for some basic components of financial revitalization such as:

- Extensive cost-cutting measures.
- Use of outside consultants.
- Enhancing long-range planning.

Some successful cost-cutting measures that one hospital used involved the controlled reduction of full-time equivalents and better management of patient length of stay. Reducing the length of stay led to fewer beds utilized and therefore resulted in less nursing care hours. Other cost-reducing measures involved benefits, management payouts, the downsizing of critical care beds, and renegotiated contracts for hospital-based physicians.

Consultant's Role

The consultant's role is to facilitate organizational change. When an organization is in a financial repositioning mode, emotions run high. Because consultants are not intimately involved in the people and the problems, they can be more objective and behave as a catalyst to accomplish tough changes. See figure 4.9 for suggestions on coping with change mandates. Consultants provide focus to cost-reduction and revenue enhancement practices. They promote a turnaround attitude and challenge management to accomplish repositioning in a timely fashion.

Figure 4.9   Coping with 4 phases of change*

Major changes are rarely taken like a Tarzan swing from one tree to another—smoothly, with a triumphal whoop.

Instead, employees usually feel as if they're on a roller coaster, being carried along on dips and rises at a frightening speed.

Change often scares people at first because it is perceived as a threat or a danger.

But, as time passes, they get used to the new state of affairs, and in so doing, begin to see its opportunities.

Understanding this common "down then up" sequence of reactions helps organizations to implement change.

Reaction to change is comparable, say consultants Cynthia Scott and Dennis Jaffe, to stages identified by psychologist Elizabeth Kubler-Ross in her work with the dying. Indeed, many changes may be considered "little deaths."

When your organization must undergo change, watch for these phases:

1. **Denial.** Denial can be observed as an initial *lack of reaction* to the change; it doesn't sink in right away. Although there's a sense of loss among employees, productivity continues for a while, causing managers to believe the transition has been accomplished.

   This is especially true if motivational speakers have pushed employees to make the "Tarzan Swing" to the new state of affairs. But a backswing comes in the form of productivity loss, as the change becomes real.

   At this point management must recognize that employees' resistance is normal, and the organization itself must respond to it.

2. **Resistance.** In the resistance phase strong feelings about the change emerge, such as self-doubt, anger, depression, anxiety, frustration, or uncertainty.

   Productivity slips, and people are often upset and negative. Some want to leave the organization.

   Employees must be allowed to express negativity safely to weather this phase. Group rituals such as award ceremonies and celebration parties help people share their experiences and thus weather the passage.

   People will reach low points on the change cycle at different rates, but eventually most will shift to the up curve.

3. **Exploration.** During the exploration phase, people draw upon their internal resources and creativity to figure out their new responsibilities and to visualize their future.

   This can be a creative, exciting time when people take on the change as an adventure and form powerful new bonds with their fellow "pioneers."

4. **Commitment.** At this point, people are ready to make stable, long-range plans and to act on them. They're willing to recreate their mission, their roles, and their expectations. This phase usually lasts until the next cycle of change begins.

Without change, organizations stagnate. At any given time, people in your unit will be in one of these phases of change, and you need to be sensitive to which phase they are experiencing.

---

*Cynthia D. Scott and Dennis T. Jaffe, *Managing Organizational Change*, Crisp Publications, 95 First St., Los Altos, CA 94022. As adapted by the Pryor Report Vol.9(1):6, 1993.

While financial innovations are working towards the turnaround process, a critical long-range strategic planning program is essential for the future success of the hospital. A firm groundwork for the hospital's future is necessary to protect against short-term fixes and to ensure continued cost effective management practices.

Eliminating Programs and Services

The strategic planning process should also have a formalized method of monitoring and evaluating services so that the winners and losers can be easily identified. Strategic planning is more than an exercise in construction managment; it is a unified effort to coordinate operations, finance, and marketing. As reimbursement tightens up, more hospitals are taking a critical look at low margin services. (See Figure 4.10) More careful and prudent scrutinization of hospital services involves financial and operational screening that can lead to exit strategies. When it is determined that a service should be eliminated, it should be because it has failed to meet multiple success criteria. (See Figure 4.11)

The Cost/Benefit Analysis

The cost/benefit analysis provides the basis for sound decision making by identifying actual costs of present operations and the estimated costs of any proposed changes. By comparing the two sets of costs, one can determine the extent of tangible and intangible benefits and the range of risks and opportunities that could present themselves. The final feature of the cost/benefit exercise is the development of an action plan for realizing new benefits and controlling program expenses. Through the analysis process the raw data is gathered that supports the decision making and provides the cues for a plan of continuous monitoring and assessment of performance.

A cost/benefit study is a must for evaluating any new service or venture. The process is especially applicable for developing propos-

Figure 4.10 Profit Margins for Some Healthcare Programs*

High Profit
Organ Transplants
Cardiovascular Services
Neurosciences
Oncology
General Surgery

Low Profit
Rehabilitation
Employee Wellness
Community Screening
Obstetrics
Behavioral Medicine

*Adapted from: Greene, Jay. "A Strategy for Cutting Back." *Modern Healthcare* 1989; 19:33-29.

Figure 4.11 Exit Strategy Criteria*

		Reinvest Yes/No	Divest Yes/No
1.	Has the service performed according to the business plan?		
2.	Has the service passed an 18-month trial period?		
3.	Do other similar programs exist that are profitable?		
4.	Has the program met its goals for units of service?		
5.	Has third party payer reimbursement performed as expected?		
6.	Are fixed costs too high?		
7.	Do collateral benefits exist to maintain the service?		
8.	Does the program have unique features that offer a competitive advantage in the market place?		
9.	Does the service exist in a mature market?		
10.	What turnaround tactics could be employed to improve financial performance?		

*Adapted from the Society for Healthcare Planning and Marketing. American Hospital Association.

als for resolving problems. The following steps can be used in designing an action plan for the reassessment of an existing service:

1. Identify the actual expenses of the existing program.
2. Identify the restraints on the present system.
3. Identify the strongest features of current operations.
4. Determine what a new or revised program will cost.
5. Describe how a new or revised program would be better than the old.
6. Describe the changes necessary to accommodate new program goals.
7. Design an action plan to accomplish program changes.
8. Conduct a detailed review of new benefits realized.

Types of Benefits

There are numerous benefits that may be identified as part of a well-performed cost/benefit analysis. Benefits generally fall into two categories: tangible and intangible. Tangible benefits may be further divided into economic and noneconomic. A tangible economic benefit is quantified in terms of dollars. Elimination of a full-time equivalent is a tangible economic benefit. (See Figure 4.12) A tangible noneconomic benefit would be an improvement in the quality of patient care. Intangible benefits are not easily converted to

Figure 4.12 Tangible Economic Benefits

People
- FTE Reduction
- FTE Enhancement

Supplies
- Inventory Reductions
- Better Utilization

Equipment
- Energy Efficient
- Increased Productivity

Purchased Services
- Controlled Maintenance Costs
- Fewer Temporaries

Revenue Improvements
- Bad Debt Reduction
- Shortened Days in Accounts Receivable
- Late and Lost Charges

---

dollars. An improvement in employee morale could lead to reductions in sick leave and improved productivity, and these changes can be converted to dollars. Intangible benefits usually have an indirect relationship to the programs and, therefore, are difficult to quantify in dollar value.

Summary

A major candidate at hospitals for a cost/benefit study is the radiology department. Other departments that would yield substantial savings opportunities include:

- Admitting.
- Business office.
- Cardiovascular services.
- Materials management.
- Laboratory.
- Pharmacy.
- Rehabilitative therapies.
- Respiratory care.
- Nursing.

The two primary products of the well executed cost/benefit exercise are the identification of savings opportunities and the development of an action plan to realize those savings.

4.6 LICENSURE OF RADIOLOGIC PROFESSIONALS

Licensure is an attempt to ensure that the healthcare professional will achieve and maintain an acceptable level of practice. It attempts to establish a national standard of excellence for radiologic technologists and represents the profession's view of what minimal standards of practice should be. Licensure will not guarantee excellence, but it will ensure at least a basic competency level in clinical practice.

In 1991, twenty-five states and Puerto Rico had enacted licensure laws. (See Figure 4.13) Ten states and the District of Columbia either had enabling legislation or legislative proposals in progress. (See Figure 4.14)

Figure 4.13 States With Licensure Laws

Arizona	Louisiana	Tennessee
California	Maine	Texas
Delaware	Maryland	Utah
Florida	Massachusetts	Vermont
Hawaii	Montana	Washington
Illinois	Nebraska	West Virginia
Indiana	New Jersey	Wyoming
Iowa	New Mexico	Puerto Rico (Commonwealth)
Kentucky	Oregon	

Figure 4.14 Other Legislative Activity

States with Proposed Legislation

Arkansas	Missouri
Colorado	North Carolina
Kansas	Pennsylvania
Michigan	Rhode Island
Mississippi	District of Columbia (federal district)

States with Enabling Legislation
Virginia
South Carolina

Individual states have been licensing radiologic technologists since the mid 1960s. The American Registry of Radiologic Technologists (ARRT) cooperated early with several states that wished to recognize the ARRT examination and certificate for licensure purposes. In 1979, the ARRT allowed the use of the ARRT examination for testing at the state level. The exam was used for state credentialing purposes only; passing the examination did not imply ARRT certification. Approximately 20 states use the ARRT examination for state licensure purposes to date. In 1983, several states requested the ARRT to develop limited scope of practice examinations.

Development of Limited Licensure

There is an examination for the limited scope of practice in radiography for licensing states under appropriate contractual arrangements with the American Registry of Radiologic Technologists (ARRT). The ARRT was founded in 1922 when the Radiological Society of North America, with support from other radiological societies, established the original organization called the American Registry of Radiological Technicians. In 1936, the registry was incorporated as The American Registry of X-ray Technicians. By 1962 growth in the field of radiologic technology was such that examination and certification in nuclear medicine technology and radiation therapy technology began. At that time, another name change occurred and the organization became the American Registry of Radiologic Technologists. In 1977, the registry adopted the term "radiographer" to replace the previous term "x-ray technologist."

The purposes of the registry include encouraging the study and elevating the standards of radiologic technology, as well as the examining and certifying of eligible candidates. The ARRT provides certification in three disciplines of radiologic technology. Those disciplines are: 1) **radiography**: the radiographer is primarily responsible for applying ionizing radiation to demonstrate portions of the human body on a radiograph, fluoroscopic screen, or other imaging modalities to assist the physician in the diagnosis of disease and injury; 2) **nuclear medicine technology**: the nuclear medicine technologist uses radioactive materials in specialized studies of body organs and/or laboratory analysis to assist the physician in the diagnosis of disease and injury; and 3) **radiation therapy technology**: the radiation therapy technologist uses ionizing radiation-producing equipment to administer therapeutic doses of radiation as prescribed by the physician for the treatment of disease.

As mentioned earlier, in addition to the three disciplines of certification already described, the registry also administers the examination for the limited scope of practice in radiography. The limited scope of practice in radiography examination was developed by the ARRT for use by states desiring to license operators on a limited basis.

The purpose of the examination for the limited scope of practice in radiography is to assess the knowledge and cognitive skills necessary to perform radiography of either the extremities or the chest. The content specifications of the examination represent some of the specifications developed for the general radiographer. It is the philosophy of the ARRT that the same knowledge and cognitive skills underlying the intelligent performance of extremity or chest radiography be the same for the limited licensee as for the entry-level staff radiographer. The first limited scope of practice examinations in radiography were administered in 1986 for chest and extremity radiography.

Pros and Cons

Those who strongly support licensure are convinced that there are vast numbers of unqualified operators of ionizing radiation-producing equipment in clinical practice today. These unqualified technologists jeopardize the safety of the public because it is assumed a lesser level of clinical competency results in increased radiation exposure and contributes to misdiagnosis due to inadequately performed studies.

Supporters also believe that licensure raises the stature of technologists and contributes in the long run to radiologic technologists being recognized as professionals. Indirectly, licensure contributes to the process of establishing radiologic technology as a profession by influencing salary levels and impacting the number of persons who may practice in the field. Licensure also insures some continuing competency among practitioners by requiring (in some states) continuing education, thus, technologists will maintain and improve their skills.

There are those who oppose licensure for a variety of reasons. Many of those opposing a licensure process argue the points raised by supporters. Chiefly, it is argued that licensure creates unnecessary bureaucracy and fees ranging from $10 to $50 annually. Licensure increases consumer healthcare costs by driving up wages and adding the expense of continuing education. The legislative process is costly, inefficient, and ineffective. Usually unqualified technologists already working when a law is enacted are grandfathered into the system.

4.7   JOINT VENTURES

Congress is seeking ways to curb the escalating costs of healthcare and looking closely at arrangements that appear to contribute to unnecessary expenses. Business arrangements between care providers and referring physicians to those providers are being scrutinized by the federal government. These joint ventures are the subject of safe harbor regulations promulgated by the Department of Health and Human Services (HHS) Office of the Inspector General (OIG). Safe harbor discussions which will follow in this review of joint ventures were placed into effect on July 29, 1991. Congress requires the OIG to define permissible conduct under the law through the Medicare and

Medicaid Patient and Program Protection Act of 1987. The new regulations discourage overutilization of diagnostic and therapeutic procedures in an effort to control Medicare costs. Congress also believes that the new regulations will increase competition in the healthcare marketplace and expand freedom of choice for the patient. These safe harbor regulations are subject to change by the legislature; so for that reason, any plans to structure a joint venture involving physicians should be carried out after careful consideration of current laws.

Proponents of joint venturing will quickly concede that it is not necessarily a quick cure or sure-fire path to financial turnaround. However, well conceived and carefully executed joint ventures can help hospitals improve their financial position, enter new markets, and enhance physician relationships. The possibilities for physician joint ventures are wide open; outpatient surgery centers, diagnostic imaging centers, and medical office buildings are the most common examples of these partnerships. Hospitals select physicians as joint venture partners because the healthcare industry is physician driven. Physicians have control of medical management of the patient; therefore, they have the greatest opportunity to control costs. Any imaging center manager will tell you that physician partners will create operating efficiencies. They are motivated to conserve costs because their return on their investment is simply a calculation of excess funds after expenses.

Forms of Joint Ventures

Joint ventures may take a number of different forms, ranging from simple contracts to complicated partnerships. Regardless of form, joint ventures need to be planned very carefully. Particular attention needs to be payed to who the participants are, what the risks entail for the financial investor, and the tax implications involved. Also, operational issues such as licensing and credentialing, reimbursement, and liability need to be managed.

There are advantages and disadvantages to the various forms of joint venture arrangements. The **contractual** model creates no new legal entity. It is merely a series of contracts. Without an integration of management structure, the arrangement is very flexible because participants are not governed by a common board of directors. The **entity** model describes a jointly-owned corporation or general partnership. The creation of this separate entity gives the joint venture a vehicle to conduct business. It also creates a board of directors to manage the affairs of the corporation. The general partnership is the most frequently used ownership structure for freestanding imaging centers. In this model, the general partner holds the greatest financial interest and usually has operational responsibility. In the **invest-ment** model joint venture, the investors take a passive role. A limited partner has a liability that is no greater than the dollar value of the investment and has no management responsibility or control. The limited partnership plan is considered to be the best way to strengthen referral relationships with physicians in your community.

Tax considerations are a major concern when forming a joint venture arrangement. Care should be taken to insure that the way the joint venture is structured will not affect the tax exempt status of the hospital which is usually the general partner. The Medicare/Medicaid Anti-Fraud and Abuse Statute and safe harbor regulations dictate the formation and operation of joint ventures. Because most joint ventures are formed by hospitals and their referring physicians, a legal review of the proposed structure of the new corporation should guide the venture into a safe harbor.

HHS Safe Harbor Regulations

Safe harbor provisions for limited or general partnerships owning imaging centers are specific and require that all investors comply with the regulatory standards. (See Figure 4.15) The safe harbor provisions must be an "all or none" situation; that is, all investors must comply or no safe harbor protection will apply to any investor in the project. The safe harbors that outline healthcare-related business activities that are protected from civil or criminal prosecution under Section 1128(b) of the Social Security Act (commonly known as the Medicare and Medicaid Anti-kickback Statute) are briefly explained below:

1. No more than 40 percent of the investment entity can be owned by anyone in a position to make referral or do any business with the entity. These passive investors cannot refer business that will result in greater than 40 percent of the venture's gross revenues.

2. Those persons not in a position to perform services for the venture or make referrals to it, must be given equal opportunity to invest in the entity. This category of investor must total at

Figure 4.15   Major Features of the Safe-Harbor Regulations*

The government's new safe-harbor regulations are designed to define what physician joint ventures are acceptable. Following are the 10 major features of the regulations:

1. No more than 40% of joint-venture investors may be capable of referring patients, and no more than 40% of total revenues can come from such referrals. Investors can't be required to refer patients, nor can they be given better dividends, services, or terms than non-referring investors.

2. Physicians may invest in large, publicly traded companies (such as drug corporations) when a company's assets are registered with the Securities and Exchange Commission and are in excess of $50 million, provided physicians are offered no more than the same services, interest, and dividends as the general public.

3. Physicians who are in a position to refer patients to health-care facilities may receive payments for space or equipment rentals in those facilities, if the facts are put in writing, with the agreement to cover at least a year, and if payments reflect the fair market value of the rentals and do not include payment for referrals.

4. Referring physicians are forbidden from receiving fees for providing consulting, managing, or personal services for a business entity, unless the details are put in writing, with the agreement to last for at least a year, and with the stipulation that the fee does not exceed the value of the services provided.

5. Doctor-to-doctor buyouts are protected if the seller leaves the practice and stops referring patients to the buyer for at least a year from the date of sale. There is no protection if the health-care entity buys a practice and the doctor becomes an employee of the facility.

6. Physicians' referral services are protected if fees charged to the doctors are based on operating costs and not referrals. Also, the service must disclose its relationship to the doctors referred.

7. Warranties for medical equipment are not considered illegal business inducements if they meet Federal Trade Commission standards.

8. Doctors may accept coupons, rebates, and discounts on purchases if such benefits do not represent cash payments for buying a particular product or a bundled arrangement where one item is discounted in exchange for the physicians' agreement to buy other goods or services.

9. Physicians may pay bona fide employees-as the term is defined by the Internal Revenue Service-in any fashion they choose.

10. Vendors offering rebates to group-purchasing entities that negotiate for physicians must limit their rebates to less than 3% of the value of the goods or services purchased. And this information must be disclosed to the doctors in writing.

---

*Adapted from Imaging Economics. Vol. 1, No. 1, March 1992. p. 7. "How safe are your harbors?"

least 60 percent of all the investors. These first two safe harbor regulations have come to be known as the "60-40" rules.

3. The terms on which any investor is invited to participate in the venture cannot be based on a past or future volume of referrals.

4. Investors may not use funds borrowed from or guaranteed by the entity to buy an interest in the venture. Further, return on investment must be strictly proportional to investment and not adjusted in any way to reflect referral activity.

There is no "grandfathering" in of any old deals that may have been made prior to the publication of these new rules. However, the OIG will take into serious consideration any evidence of a diligent attempt to restructure old agreements to comply with new safe harbor provisions.

Space and Equipment Rental

For radiology managers who may be in a position to negotiate issues of space and equipment rental, it is important to know that safe harbor provisions are essentially the same as for investment entities. There are five conditions that must be met for rental agreements to be considered legal. The five conditions are:

1. There must be a signed written lease agreement.
2. The lease must specify the property involved.
3. The lease must spell out any limitations to access of space or equipment.
4. The lease must be for at least a year.
5. The rent must be set in advance at fair market value and not tied to volume or the value of any referrals.

Other Safe Harbor Rules

Other safe harbor rules affect areas such as personal services and managmeent contracts, sales of practices, referral services, warranties, discounts, and waivers of coinsurance and deductibles. It is advisable to consult expert advice for an interpretation of safe harbor requirements in any area of investment practice and relationships anticipated with physicians. Failure to comply with new safe harbor provisions doesn't mean that current arrangements are illegal, but knowing the rules and functioning under their guidance will certainly help avoid prosecution for fraud and abuse.

Managing the Joint Venture Process

Joint venturing a service, like a diagnostic imaging center, can serve as an effective means of raising capital and sharing the financial risks with many investors. Joint ventures were relatively rare a decade ago and, despite cautions from the federal government, are widespread and accepted as good business strategies today.

Managing the process of a joint venture can likely fall on the shoulders of the radiology manager. Every joint venture will be different. There is no boilerplate process to guide the novice through the conundrum of local circumstances, wants, and needs. There are, however, many issues that are common to every joint venture project. Joint venturing is a process of creative decision making that springs from a planning procedure. The early plans of the joint venture will not be cast in stone. Early written planning documents will involve over-all goals, preliminary plans, and test pro formas. All of these written planning documents will provide the parties in the venture with a basis for discussions. It will be these early planning discussions that will set the agenda for issues, contingencies, and financial concerns which will make up the final written partnership agreement. A number of questions need to be asked and the answers to those questions will fashion the form of a mutually satisfying final document for the joint venture.

Legal counsel with experience in joint venture agreements must be obtained at the very beginning of the process. There will be many individuals involved in the new entity; often each participant will have their own attorney.

Some of the legal issues which need to be addressed early are:

- Who will own the joint venture?
- Who will manage its affairs?
- How will company policies be developed?
- What will occur in the event of death, resignation, incompetency, disability, or retirement of any principals?
- How long will the contract be in effect?

- How can changes be made to the structure of the venture?
- Under what circumstances can the venture agreement be dissolved?
- Will the venture meet all existing local, state, and federal laws governing such arrangements?
- What are the insurance issues?
- Have all tax considerations been covered?

Financial Concerns of Joint Venture

1. What will be the method of funding?
2. How will equity in the project be distributed?
3. When will earnings be disbursed?
4. What are the tax implications for each participant?
5. Will legal changes in the future affect the finances?

Operational Issues for Joint Ventures

1. Is there a written business plan that covers marketing?
2. Who will be responsible for daily operations?
3. How will the success of the venture be measured?
4. Will the venture have the flexibility to expand for a growing market?

Conclusion

This safe harbor discussion has been elementary and meant to alert the radiology manager to the many considerations that must be taken into account when planning for a joint venture. The final rules of Section 14 of the Medicare/Medicaid Patient and Program Protection Act of 1987 identify various payment practices which are protected from criminal and civil sanctions under anti-kickback statutes. The statutes provide civil and criminal penalties to those who knowingly violate them. A violation may be prosecuted and involve fines of up to $25,000, imprisonment, and exclusion of participation in the medicare program as a provider for up to five years.

Joint venture participants should understand that noncompliance with any safe harbor does not automatically imply guilt of fraud and abuse. As with all law, ambiguities result from interpretation of the statutes. When forming a joint venture in the future, be sure that referrals are not encouraged in any way by promise of benefits to the referrer.

4.8 THE JOINT COMMISSION ON ACCREDITATION OF HEALTHCARE ORGANIZATIONS

Meeting JCAHO Standards

The Joint Commission on Accreditation of Healthcare Organizations (JCAHO) is an ambitious and dynamic organization that provides a means for healthcare professionals to achieve and maintain high quality healthcare services. Currently, it accredits more than 6,000 acute-care hospitals across the United States. It is a private, voluntary, nonprofit organization that is in the business of accreditation.

History

Concerns about improving healthcare found organized beginnings early in the twentieth century. The JCAHO is a descendant of the hospital standardization program that was established by the American College of Surgeons in 1918. The ACS encouraged the formation of a format for recording medical records. It recognized the need for a system of standardization, identifying institutions supporting the highest ideals of medicine and patient care. In 1951, five major associations of North American medicine and hospitals joined to create the JCAHO, whose sole purpose was to encourage the voluntary attainment of uniformly high standards of hospital care. Its initial founding members were the ACS, the American College of Physicians, the American Hospital Association, the American Medical Association, and the Canadian Medical Association. In 1969, the Canadian Council on Hospital Accreditation was founded and joined in the endeavor of the JCAHO.

The JCAHO adopted standards developed by the ACS during its 35 years of operation. Hospitals meeting ACS standards were accredited by the JCAHO. In 1952, the JCAHO began a careful review of the standards and also began granting accreditation to other hospitals seeking approval.

Between 1953 and 1965, the hospital accreditation standards were revised six times. In 1965 JCAHO standards were specifically referred to by law. Public Law 89-97 (Medicare) represented the confidence Congress had that the healthcare sector, chiefly through the efforts of the JCAHO, was able to voluntarily assess the quality of medical care being provided in the nation. The standards of the commission were specifically referred to in the law. Written into the Medicare Act was the provision that hospitals participating in the program should maintain the level of patient care that was recognized by JCAHO standards. As a result of the 1965 Medicare legislation, hospitals accredited by the JCAHO were considered to be in compliance with federal Medicare conditions of participation.

In 1966, the JCAHO board of commissioners voted to re-evaluate and rewrite hospital accreditation standards. The decision was prompted by an awareness that the nation's hospitals were eager to achieve higher levels of healthcare than were currently required. The commission wanted to attain two main objectives through this endeavor. The first was to raise and strengthen the standards to an optimal, achievable level and to assure that they were suitable to the state of the art of medical care. The second objective was to simplify and clarify the language of the standards.

Purpose of JCAHO

Throughout the more than 40 years of growth and expansion of the commission, one thing has remained unchanged—the purpose of the JCAHO.

The purpose of the JCAHO is threefold: to establish standards, conduct surveys, and award accreditation. The commission serves as an evaluator and educator rather than inspector or judge. It acts as a consultant, helping to identify both strong and weak points, and provides guidelines to assist in correcting the weaknesses. The JCAHO has become a forum through which healthcare providers and related human services can be effectively motivated toward higher levels of quality and service.

The JCAHO is not a regulatory agency of the government; it is a private, nonprofit corporation whose purpose is voluntary accreditation. The activities of the JCAHO are sometimes misunderstood because accreditation activities are confused with licensure or certification. Accreditation is based on optimal, achievable standards, which distinguishes the purpose of the JCAHO from regulatory determinations like certification. Certification usually applies to a facility's ability to operate according to minimum standards.

Development of Standards

The JCAHO standards are specifically written to contain provisions that relate to the quality of healthcare services, and in so doing, validate those services as necessary. The standards ensure that services are optimally provided. Compliance with the standards is demonstrated as measurable in a practical means and achievable in existing facilities.

Standards develop out of a desire to improve the quality of a particular facet of healthcare services. Because this desire exists on a continual basis, the development of JCAHO standards is an ongoing process. Changes in modern medical care practices and governmental regulations trigger the need to revise and develop new standards. Recently, consumer demands for accountability and the rising concern for cost containment have become important in the standards development process.

The 1992 Accreditation Manual for Hospitals is a major revision of the previous manual and an initial step towards a carefully planned transition to standards that emphasize continuous quality improvement. Reformulating the standards is one of three major initiatives that make up the JCAHO's "Agenda for Change." The other initiatives are to redesign the survey process and to develop performance measures related to the standards. The actual number of standards is shrinking; 1992 standards contained nearly a one-third reduction in total standards. The manual is more concise and much less redundant than previous editions. Many of the deleted standards have been incorporated into the new scoring guidelines. The JCAHO standards for diagnostic radiology, nuclear medicine, and radiation oncology are available to you directly from the JCAHO. It is almost certain that one or more officials in your organization have copies of the most recent edition of the *Accreditation Manual for Hospitals* and the *Scoring Guidelines*. You should always have the latest version of applicable standards in your office. The following text from the 1992 Manual and *Scoring Guidelines* is an example of the standards and their interpretations.

1. **DR.1.3.2.2** At least one qualified radiologic technologist is on duty or available when needed.

    *   **INTENT** A hospital must maintain diagnostic radiology services over a continuous 24-hour period, seven days a week. A qualified technologist should be available within approximately 30 minutes when the decision is made that a radiology (image) study is indicated.
    *   **SCORING—Score 1** At least one qualified radiologic technologist is available at all times. If the technologist is on call, response time is approximately 30 minutes from the time it has been determined that a diagnostic radiology study is indicated.

        —Score 2 Once or twice in the past year a qualified technologist has not been available at all times.

        OR

        Response time has exceeded 30 minutes on one or two occasions in the past year.

        —Score 3 A qualified technologist has not been available at all times.

        OR

        Response time has exceeded 30 minutes on more than two occasions in the past year.

        —Score 4 A qualified technologist is on duty only during daytime hours. The facility provides no coverage during evening and weekend hours.

        OR

        Response time regularly exceeds 30 minutes.

        —Score 5 A qualified technologist is not available at all times.

2. **DR.1.3.2.3** A radiologic technologist does not independently perform diagnostic fluoroscopic procedures for the purpose of interpretive fluoroscopy except for those localizing procedures approved by the director of the diagnostic radiology department/service.

- **INTENT** Only licensed independent practitioners with appropriate clinical privileges should perform and interpret diagnostic radiology studies employing fluoroscopy for visualization of function of organs (for example, upper gastrointestinal series or barium enema using contrast media).
- **SCORING—Score 1** Technologists or other nonindependent personnel perform diagnostic fluoroscopy or invasive diagnostic studies (for example, gastrointestinal studies) only under direct supervision by a qualified licensed independent practitioner who has the appropriate clinical privileges. Positioning procedures (for example, for a cholecystogram) may be performed by trained personnel if the director of radiology services has authorized qualified individuals to do so.
  —Score 5 Frequently technologists or other personnel who do not practice independently perform diagnostic fluoroscopy and/or invasive diagnostic studies without a qualified independent practitioner present who has the clinical privilege to perform the procedure.

Implementation of Standards

The JCAHO realizes that the type and size of a hospital seeking accreditation dictates the methods used to meet the standards. The standards are comprehensive and applicable to most hospitals that would seek accreditation. *Scoring Guidelines* are published by the JCAHO to assist hospitals in understanding the standards and their compliances. Total compliance with the standards is not always necessary to achieve accreditation, but substantial, overall compliance must be demonstrated by an institution to meet the approval of surveyors. The accreditation decision is a judgement by the commission of whether reasonable compliance exists. The commission understands that complete compliance with every standard is rarely attained. The scoring guidelines serve as a guide for hospitals to ensure that efficient patient care is provided according to the prescribed standards. The standards are not intended to restrict the practice of medicine but, instead, allow for variations that still indicate quality in the delivery of healthcare.

Scoring Guidelines

Scoring guidelines should not be confused with standards. The standards state the expectation that must be met in order to achieve compliance. The scoring guidelines set the parameters for surveyor judgement by specifying levels of meeting the standard. The scoring guidelines offer the most common way that the intent of the standard may be met.

Scoring guidelines were originally developed to help surveyors in being consistent in interpretation of standards. The publication of these scoring guidelines has greatly improved the readiness of facilities for surveyor visits. The scoring guidelines, for the most part, have taken the mystery out of compliance with standards. In essence, the game has become much easier to play now that everyone knows the rules!

Preparing for the Site Visit

The anticipation associated with an upcoming survey visit results in a rush of preparation shortly before the date of inspection. Don't let this last minute rite of preparation occur in your facility. While a certain amount of final preparation may be necessary, the process of "getting ready" for the joint commission should begin 18 months before the visit. This long lead time is mainly to assure compliance with any ongoing monitoring for at least a year in duration.

A **focused preparation process** should be in place no later than eight months prior to your survey. The purpose of this focused preparation process is to determine the current degree of compliance to standards, recognize and correct any deficiencies, and avoid last minute scrambles for required documentation. This focused preparation process is a four step procedure:

1. Orientation to the radiology standards.
2. Self-assessment and evaluation.
3. Mock survey.
4. Re-evaluation.

The preparatory process should be completed a month prior to the scheduled survey. A conference with all involved individuals would be held at that time to discuss plans to make the actual day of the survey flow smoothly. At this time each person will know his role during the surveyor interview; one individual will serve as overall coordinator and host to the Joint Commission surveyor. See figure 4.16 for a suggested calendar for JCAHO preparation.

Step 1: Orientation to the Radiology Standards

The current *Accreditation Manual for Hospitals* and the corresponding scoring guidelines are discussed one at a time. Testing for understanding of their intents and a review of the degree of compliance that exists to the standards is conducted. Evidence of ongoing activity that demonstrates compliance for a required time frame must be documented to satisfactorily meet the requirements of the standards. A surveyor will sometimes give credit to a corrective plan when it is discovered that substantial compliance hasn't existed. The corrective plan should reflect understanding of the intent of the standard and a mechanism to assure the standard will be met.

Step 2: Self-Assessment and Evaluation

The self-assessment process devises and implements corrective action plans. One approach to self-assessment is to identify individuals responsible for the review of certain standards. The self-assessment with the use of the scoring guidelines should begin immediately following Step 1. The self-assessment step will take six to eight weeks to complete. As individuals complete the self-assessment, they will determine the degree of compliance with the standards. Deficient areas will be addressed with corrective plans and targeted completion dates. Periodic plan of action reports (every two weeks) will monitor progress towards resolving deficiencies.

Figure 4.16 Calendar for JCAHO Preparation

18 Months	8 Months	1 Month	Survey Day
	Steps 1-4		
Preparation process begins. Hospital designates JCAHO Preparation Coordinator.	Department JCAHO Preparation Coordinator begins focused process.	All preparation is completed. Final enhancing details are put in place.	

Step 3: Mock Survey

If you work in a hospital, it is probable that part of the institution's preparation for a survey visit will be a hospital mock survey. The mock survey will usually be conducted by an outside agency such as the state hospital association or a consultant group. Radiology will be visited by mock surveyors if your hospital avails itself to this self-evaluation opportunity.

A radiology department mock survey is part of your focused preparation process. As coordinator of the preparatory process, you will serve as a mock surveyor along with one or two other individuals who must be knowledgeable of JCAHO standards. Deficiencies discovered at this time will need immediate attention.

Step 4: Re-evaluation

The final stage of JCAHO advanced preparation will be to zero in on those areas found to be deficient in steps 2 and 3. If the corrective action plans were followed, a "clean" survey visit from the JCAHO can be anticipated. If this final evaluation still identifies areas that need corrective action, close monitoring to clear up remaining deficiencies must be strictly adhered to.

While a process of focused preparation is going to be beneficial, a climate of ongoing evaluation is much better. An ongoing mechanism to evaluate compliance with JCAHO standards is the safest policy to follow. A system of quarterly review of selected JCAHO standards associated with the department quality assessment and improvement plan is a convenient way to keep an edge on compliance with the standards.

What the JCAHO Will Be Looking for

The radiology department manager is responsible for preparing or providing certain **administrative manuals and documents**. The manuals should be approved, reviewed, and signed annually by the medical director and cosigned by the appropriate administrative official in your organization (usually your boss). Each manual should have a table of contents, and the department's name and the manual's title should be displayed on the front and spine of its binder. The following list of manuals should be available for the surveyor to review. As the manager you must be familiar with the contents of each manual. You don't want to fumble around with sometimes lengthy volumes for a policy or piece of documentation the surveyor has asked to see.

1. Department policy and procedure manual.
2. Quality assessment and improvement manual.
3. Infection control manual.
4. Safety manual (to include radiation safety).
5. Hazardous waste procedures.
6. Emergency preparedness manual/hospital disaster plan.
7. Continuing education manual.
8. Administrative manual.
9. Human resources policies and procedures.
10. Job descriptions, purpose, mission, and organizational charts.

There will be a **general plant and technology safety** tour of the hospital. Usually the administrative member of the survey team inspects plant technology and safety. During the tour of the radiology department, the following safety areas may be addressed in detail:

- **General safety**
    1. Locked medicine carts
    2. Areas free of clutter
    3. Safety policies and procedures
- **Hazardous materials and waste management**
    1. Material safety data sheets
    2. Documentation of employee inservices
    3. Infectious waste handling
- **Emergency preparedness**
    1. Fire plan
    2. Disaster plan
    3. Contingency plan
    4. Will ask employees their role in each
- **Equipment management**
    1. Written records must exist on all equipment
    2. Equipment user training is documented
    3. When problems are identified, actions are taken to resolve them

- **Utilities management**
    1. Employees must know their contingency plans in the event of a utility failure
    2. Know the location of emergency cutoffs
    3. When problems are identified, actions are taken to resolve them
- **Life safety**
    1. Fire extinguishing equipment in place and inspected
    2. Evaluation routes posted
    3. Employees must know the hospital smoking policy
    4. Corridors must be clear
    5. Exit lights must be illuminated
    6. Stairwells and equipment rooms must be free of storage
    7. Doors must not have impediments from closing and latching

The physician surveyor will place a great deal of emphasis on **quality assessment and improvement** activities. This area of quality assurance will need to have an established track record that is obvious in your documentation. A program cannot demonstrate that it has been effective if it has not been in operation for at least a year. Your compliance with JCAHO requirements for continuous quality improvement may be ascertained by your ability to respond to the following questions:

1. Does your department monitor and evaluate the quality and appropriateness of patient care services it provides and resolve identified problems?
    - Is the monitoring and evaluation process planned and systematically carried out?
    - Is the physician director of your department responsible for assuring that the monitoring and evaluation process is being carried out?
2. Have you accurately described the scope of service you provide, including the patient population, diagnoses, conditions, and procedures performed?
3. Have you identified important aspects of care or services?
    - Do these include high-volume procedures, such as computerized tomography studies?

- Do these include aspects of care that are problem prone, such as studies involving the use of intravenous contrast media?
- Do these include high-risk procedures, such as angioplasty studies and cardiac studies of compromised patients?

4. In conducting monitoring and evaluation activities, do you use indicators that specify the activities, events, or outcomes to be measured? For example, "The radiologist's reports are accurate."

5. In conducting monitoring and evaluation activities, do you use criteria to evaluate the indicators? For example, "The radiologist's report agrees with pathology reports, endoscopy findings, or pulmonary function studies."

6. In conducting monitoring and evaluation activities, do you collect data and make sure variations from criteria are peer reviewed?

7. When unjustified variations from criteria are identified, is corrective action taken to resolve the problem?

8. Is there a follow-up of the corrective action to assure the problem has been permanently resolved and an acceptable level of quality achieved and maintained?

9. Are the findings from your quality assurance activities reported to appropriate services and committees, as described in the hospital-wide quality assurance plan?

- Are the findings from quality assurance activities used in the appraisal and reappraisal of practitioners' competence and in the delineation of their clinical privileges?*

New Areas of Survey Concentration

Patient, family education. Hospital care-givers must provide to patients and their families, including significant others, specific information relevant to their health care needs. They must include information on the safe and effective use of medication and medical equipment; instruction on potential drug-food interactions and counseling on modified diets; and how and when to obtain further treatment if needed.

---

*Buff, Hugh. "Preparing for the JCAH Survey." *Administrative Radiology.* 6(7):28-32, 1987.

Surveyors will not expect to see new patient education departments, committees or services. Hospitals also have leverage to determine which professionals within the hospital will provide this
education to the patient and family. Radiology nurses will need to
focus on discharge instructions following interventional procedures,
instructions for special preparations, and radiation therapy.

Consistent orientations. The *AMH* chapter on orientation, training and education of staff members emphasizes the importance of
preparing them for their job responsibilities, as well as the need to
maintain professional competence through well-planned education
activities. The standards are not applicable to medical staff members, but
do apply to employees working in medical staff departments/services.

The focus here is to provide a "coordinated orientation of new staff".

Surveyors will be looking to see that all staff members undergo an
orientation program that includes information on:

- Mission, governance, and policies and procedures of the
  organization and the department/service
- An individual's job description
- Performance expectations
- The organization's plant, technology, and safety management
  functions and the individual's safety responsibilities
- The organization's infection-control program and the individual's
  role in the prevention of infection
- The organization's program for quality assessment and
  improvement activities.

Education should help employees maintain and improve the
required level of knowledge and skill to perform their jobs. Specifically,
surveyors will be looking for continuing education programs based on:

- Patient population served
- Type and nature of care provided by the hospital and the
  department/service
- Individual staff member needs
- Information from quality assessment and improvement activities,
  performance appraisals, review by peers activities, safety
  management programs and infection-control activities.
- Needs generated by advances made in health care management
  and health care science and technology

Employees must be competent in the use of equipment; the prevention of contamination and transfer of infection; cardiopulmonary resuscitation and other lifesaving measures.

Credentials, personnel files and training schedules are examples of the types of documentation surveyors will expect to see in order to evaluate compliance with these standards.

Department directors. Responsibilities of department/service directors address leadership responsibilities.

Surveyors will examine how well department directors carry out such duties as coordinating department goals with those of the hospital; coordinating their departments with others; developing and implementing policies and procedures; determining the qualifications and competence of staff members; assessing and improving the quality of care provided by the department; and recommending the need for such resources as space, training, personnel, expertise or financial support.

Surveyors will also check to see that every surveyed hospital has a plan in place for how its leaders will meet the following quality improvement standards:

- Set priorities for quality improvement activities
- Allocate resources for improvement activities
- Train staff members regarding quality improvement
- Foster better communication and coordination of quality improvement activities within the hospital
- Analyze the effectiveness of their contributions to quality improvement.*

Appendix A—JCAHO

How to Conduct Yourself During the Survey Interview

8 Points

1. Use the opportunity to make a good impression verbally and nonverbally.
2. Be thoroughly familiar with your section of the manual.

---

* Koska, M.T., JCAHO Introduces three new areas of survey concentration. *Hospitals.* Oct. 5, 1992, pp. 62-64.

3. Be certain that any previous recommendations have been corrected.
4. Be prepared with the materials the surveyor expects to see.
5. Have policies and procedures up-to-date and properly reviewed and signed-off on.
6. Answer questions directly. Do not offer additional information.
7. Ask to be shown standards and interpretations for recommendations you feel are unreasonable. Ask for advice on how the standard may be met.
8. Don't gossip. Stay focused on your area of responsibility.

Appendix B—JCAHO

Pre–JCAHO Survey Tips

Do's

- Know the JCAHO standards for your areas and any recent proposed changes to the standards.
- Make sure your area is neat and clean on the day of the survey. It should be free of clutter, storage material, and stacks of paper.
- Have ample numbers of chairs available or schedule a convenient conference room that will accommodate four individuals.
- Be familiar with hazardous material, MSDS forms, right-to-know procedures, and procedures regarding safety, disaster preparedness, and infection control.
- Rehearse the use of your policy and procedure manual, the documentation of inservice education, and your QA process.
- Review your performance appraisal system, reacquainting yourself with its key components.
- Be prepared to use terms such as "quality improvement, indications, thresholds, opportunities for improvement," and "actions and evidence of effectiveness or follow-up."
- Ask the surveyor how your area fared. Specifically ask if there are any Type 1 recommendations. If there are any, write them down and forward them to administration immediately.

Don'ts

- Don't antagonize or challenge either the JCAHO surveyors or the standards themselves. The surveyors did not set the standards. Defend without being defensive!

- Don't try to monopolize the conversation. Don't run on or try to embellish the answer. Answer the surveyor's question directly and concisely.
- Don't be too quick to volunteer unnecessary information such as: "The last manager didn't really have his act together," or "We haven't found any significant problems yet, but we continue to monitor."
- Don't bring up past surveys or past management of the departments. These remarks often sound like excuses for poor institutional performance and rarely, if ever, evoke sympathy from the surveyor.

Appendix C—JCAHO

		MANAGEMENT POLICY
	COMPANY/LOCATION	STANDARD PROCEDURE

SUBJECT	DEPARTMENT	NUMBER
Mandatory Continuing Education		PAGE
TITLE	**DATE EFFECTIVE**	**DATE REVISED**
JCAHO Recommended In-Services	APPROVED BY (Signature)	APPROVED BY (Signature)

POLICY: In keeping with the hospital's commitment to provide consistent quality care, each director/manager is responsible for scheduling employee attendance at mandatory educational programs each year. Documentation of attendance will be kept in departmental education records.

PROCEDURE: 1. The department director/manager is responsible for scheduling each employee to attend mandatory programs and for documentation of such in the department education record.

    2. Department directors/managers are responsible for conducting and maintaining documentation of the departments' specific programs related to these topics annually.

RECOMMENDED EDUCATIONAL REQUIREMENTS (JCAHO):

1. Infection control.   4. Hazardous materials.

2. Fire.   5. Disaster.

3. Safety   6. Back care.

7. CPR (only when required by regulatory agencies and departmental
   policy and procedure).

            3. Department directors/managers are responsible for
   ensuring that topics specific to the operation of a
   particular department are presented in a timely
   fashion and that employees attend these programs
   appropriately.

Appendix D—JCAHO

*Glossary of JCAHO Terms**

Accreditation A determination by the Joint Commission that an eligible hospital complies substantially with applicable Joint Commission standards.

Accreditation Survey An evaluation of a hospital to assess its level of compliance with applicable standards and make determinations regarding its accreditation status. The survey includes evaluation of documentation of compliance provided by hospital personnel; verbal information concerning the implementation of standards, or examples of their implementation, that will enable a determination of compliance to be made; and on-site observations by surveyors. The survey also provides the opportunity for education and consultation to hospitals regarding standard compliance.

    survey team The group of healthcare professionals who work together to perform an accreditation survey. The basic hospital survey team consists of a physician, a nurse, and administrative surveyors. A laboratorian and other specialist surveyors (for example, a mental health surveyor) may be added to evaluate certain services provided by a hospital.

    surveyor A physician, nurse, an administrator, a laboratorian, or any other healthcare professional who meets Joint Commission

---

*Adapted from the *JCAHO Accreditation Manual for Hospitals*. 1992.

surveyor selection criteria, evaluates standard compliance, and provides education and consultation regarding standard compliance to surveyed hospitals.

Aspects of Care, important Care activities or processes that occur frequently or affect large numbers of patients; that place patients at risk of serious consequences if care is not provided correctly, if incorrect care is provided, or if correct care is not provided; and/or that tend to produce problems for patients or staff. Such activities or processes are deemed most important for purposes of monitoring and evaluation.

Cardiopulmonary Resuscitation (CPR) The administration of artificial heart and lung action in the event of cardiac and/or respiratory arrest. The two major components of cardiopulmonary resuscitation are artificial ventilation and closed-chest cardiac massage.

Clinical Privileges Authorization granted by the governing body to a practitioner to provide specific patient care services in the hospital within defined limits, based on an individual practitioner's license, education, training, experience, competence, health status, and judgement.

Compliance To act in accordance with, as in "compliance with a standard."
> **compliance level** A measure of the extent to which a hospital acts in accordance with a specified standard, including:
> > **substantial compliance** A hospital consistently meets all major provisions of a specified standard, designated by a score 1.
> > **significant compliance** A hospital meets most provisions of a standard, designated by a score 2.
> > **partial compliance** A hospital meets some of the provisions of a standard, designated by a score 3.
> > **minimal compliance** A hospital meets few of the provisions of a standard, designated by a score 4.
> > **noncompliance** A hospital fails to meet the provisions of a standard, designated by a score 5.
> > **not applicable** The standard does not apply to the hospital, designated by NA.

Continuing Education Education beyond initial professional preparation that is relevant to the type of patient care delivered in the hospital, that provides current knowledge relevant to an individual's field of practice, and that is related to findings from quality assessment and improvement activities.

Credentialing The process of the governing body granting authorization to provide specific patient care and treatment services in the hospital, within defined limits, based on an individual's license, education, training, experience, competence, health status, and judgement.

Criteria Expected level(s) of achievement against which performance or care can be evaluated.
   clinical criteria See guideline, practice and parameters, practice.
   criteria for survey eligibility Conditions necessary for hospitals to be surveyed for accreditation. The criteria address the structure, functions, and services of the hospital.

Diagnostic Radiology Services The delivery of care pertaining to the use of radiant energy for the diagnosis of disease. Standards are applied to evaluate a hospital's performance in providing diagnostic radiology care.
   medical radiation physicist, qualified An individual who is certified by the American Board of Radiology in the appropriate disciplines of radiologic physics, including diagnostic, therapeutic, and/or medical nuclear physics; or an individual who demonstrates equivalent competency in these disciplines.
   radiologic technologist, qualified An individual who is a graduate of a program in radiologic technology approved by the Council on Medical Education of the American Medical Association or who has the documented equivalent in education and training.

Emergency Preparedness Plan/Program A component of a hospital's safety management program designed to manage the consequences of natural disasters or other emergencies that disrupt the hospital's ability to provide care and treatment.

Equipment Management A component of a hospital's plant, technology, and safety management program designed to assess and control the clinical and physical risks of fixed and portable equipment used for the diagnosis, treatment, monitoring, and care of patients and of other fixed and portable electrically powered equipment.

Guideline, scoring Descriptive tool that is used to assist hospitals in their efforts to comply with Joint Commission standards and to determine degrees of compliance. Scoring guidelines are described in *Accreditation Manual for Hospitals, Vol. II.*

Intent of Standard A brief explanation of the meaning and significance of a standard.

Joint Commission on Accreditation of Healthcare Organizations An independent, not-for-profit organization dedicated to improving the quality of care in organized healthcare settings. Founded in 1951, its members are the American College of Physicians, the American College of Surgeons, the American Dental Association, the American Hospital Association, and the American Medical Association. The major functions of the Joint Commission include organizational standards development, award of accreditation decisions, and provisions of education and consultation to healthcare organizations.

Licensed Independent Practitioner Any individual who is permitted by law and by the hospital to provide patient care services without direction or supervision, within the scope of the individual's license and in accordance with individually granted clinical privileges.

Medical Staff A hospital body that has the overall responsibility for the quality of the professional services provided by individuals with clinical privileges and also the responsibility of accounting therefore to the governing body. The medical staff includes fully licensed physicians and may include other licensed individuals permitted by law and by the hospital to provide patient care services independently in the hospital. Members have delineated clinical privileges that allow them to provide patient care services independently within the scope of their clinical privileges. Members and all others with individual clinical privileges are subject to medical staff and departmental bylaws and to review as part of the hospital's quality assessment and improvement activities. Standards are applied to evaluate the quality of a hospital's medical staff performance.

Mission Statement A written expression that sets forth the purpose of a hospital or a component thereof; it usually precedes the formation of goals and objectives of the hospital or a component thereof.

Monitoring and Evaluation A process designed to help hospitals effectively use their quality assessment and improvement resources by focusing on high-priority quality-of-care issues. The process includes identification of the most important aspects of the care the hospital (or department/service) provides; use of indicators to systematically monitor these aspects of care; evaluation of the care at least when thresholds are approached or reached to identify opportunities for improvement or problems; taking action(s) to improve care or solve problems; evaluation of the effectiveness of those actions; and communicating findings through established channels.

Nuclear Medicine Services The delivery of scientific and clinical care involving the diagnostic, therapeutic (exclusive of sealed radium sources), and investigative use of radionuclides. Standards are applied to evaluate a hospital's performance in providing nuclear medicine services.

Quality Assessment The measurement of the technical and interpersonal aspects of healthcare and services and the outcomes of that care and service. Quality assessment provides information that may be used in quality improvement activities.

Quality Assessment and Improvement The ongoing activities designed to objectively and systematically evaluate the quality of patient care and services, to pursue opportunities to improve patient care and services, and to resolve identified problems. Standards are applied to evaluate the quality of a hospital's performance in conducting quality assessment and improvement activities.

Quality Improvement An approach to the continuous study and improvement of the process of providing healthcare services to meet the needs of patients and others. Synonyms and near-synonyms include continuous quality improvement (CQI), continuous improvement (CI), and total quality management (TQM).

Radiation Oncology Services Delivery of care pertaining to the use of radiation therapy for patients with tumors. Standards are applied to evaluate a hospital's performance in providing radiation oncology services.

Standard A statement of expectation that defines the structures and processes that must be substantially in place in an organization to enhance the quality of care.

Type I Recommendation A recommendation or group of recommendations that affect adversely the accreditation decision and should be addressed in the hospital's plan for improvement. Progress in resolving type I recommendations is monitored by the Joint Commission through focused surveys or written progress reports, or both, at stated times during the accreditation cycle. Failure to resolve such compliance issues within stated time frames can result in the loss of accreditation.

Type II Recommendation A recommendation or group of recommendations that are supplementary or consultative in nature and do not affect the accreditation decision. They can, however, affect that decision if not remedied by the time of the next triennial survey.

Appendix E

Life Safety Inspection

This is a list of the most common things that the fire safety inspector will be looking for when they survey a hospital. This is intended only to be a general guideline for people to use in maintaining good safety habits.

1. Obstructed corridors - items cannot be left in open public/ patient corridors for *any* reason. Some common items left in the patient corridors are:
   a. unoccupied patient beds
   b. stretchers
   c. linen carts
   d. trash carts
   e. dietary tray carts
2. Medication carts *cannot* be left unattended in corridors for *any* reason.
3. Exit lights should be illuminated at all times and visible from any place in the public corridor.
4. Doors being propped open with wedges or being held open by other items are not permitted. Doors to storage rooms, locker rooms, linen rooms, kitchens, treatment rooms, janitor closets, etc. should be closed at all times.
5. Obstructed fire extinguishers—staff must have easy access to fire extinguishers and fire hoses in any situation at any time.

6. Doors should latch properly when closed and doors with automatic closures should close and latch securely when released.
7. Exit accesses should not be blocked by any items. Employees, staff, and visitors must have direct access to all exits at any time.
8. Fire inspectors look upon clutter as being fire hazards.
9. Areas where dirty laundry or trash is stored must be secured at all times with doors being properly closed and latched.

Appendix F—Safety Profiles

Hallways, Stairs & Exit Paths

Date: _____   Location: _____

                          Surveyor: _____

YES	NO	N/A	
[ ]	[ ]	[ ]	Are all carts, wheelchairs, and/or other items in the corridors placed along the same side of the hall, or otherwise placed so that they do not create an obstacle course?
[ ]	[ ]	[ ]	Are the corridors reasonably clear of obstructions?
[ ]	[ ]	[ ]	Are any wet floors marked with CAUTION, WET FLOOR (or similar) signs?
[ ]	[ ]	[ ]	Is carpeting secure to the floor, unfrayed, free from tripping hazards, and generally in good condition?
[ ]	[ ]	[ ]	Are hard floor surfaces secure to the floor and free of tripping and slipping hazards?
[ ]	[ ]	[ ]	Are all EXIT signs illuminated?
[ ]	[ ]	[ ]	When opened and then released, do all fire doors close and latch properly?
[ ]	[ ]	[ ]	Are stairwell handrails in good condition?
[ ]	[ ]	[ ]	Are stairwell treads in good condition?
[ ]	[ ]	[ ]	Are stairwells completely clear of obstructions and any objects. (Stairwells may not be used for storage.)

Please list any comments made by staff in your area, or your own observations, which may help reduce accidents.

Fire and Disaster

Date: _____   Location: _____

                             Surveyor: _____

YES NO N/A

[ ] [ ] [ ] Are all fire alarm boxes and fire extinguishers readily identifiable and accessible?

[ ] [ ] [ ] Do staff all know the locations of at least 2 fire extinguishers in or near their work area?

[ ] [ ] [ ] Are staff in the area familiar with the location of the Disaster Manual and the Safety Manual?

[ ] [ ] [ ] Do staff in the area seem to know the proper reporting procedure if they find (or believe there may be) a fire?

FOR YOUR INFORMATION:

1. Remove persons from immediate danger.

2. Report the fire by first pulling down on the fire alarm, and then call the operator using the emergency number.

3. Extinguish the fire ONLY after the above has been done.

4. Smoke must be reported as a fire. Strange odors which may be smoke or from fire may be either reported as a fire or just phoned into the hospital operator - but don't just leave the situation go unreported...we must check out all possible fire situations.

[ ] [ ] [ ] Is NOTHING stored closer than 18 inches from the ceiling?

[ ] [ ] [ ] Are all containers of powders, liquids and gases labeled to indicate what they contain.

[ ] [ ] [ ] Did you observe anyone smoking in the corridors or other no smoking locations?

Who? (Use the back of this sheet.)

[ ]   [ ]   [ ]   Are NO SMOKING signs prominently posted wherever oxygen cylinders are present, oxygen flowmeters are plugged into the wall (whether in use or not) or oxygen is being administered?

[ ]   [ ]   [ ]   Are all wastebaskets and ashtrays in the area made of non-combustible material?

General Safety

Date: _____   Location: _____

                                   Surveyor: _____

YES NO N/A

[ ]   [ ]   [ ]   Are drawers kept closed at all times when not actually in use?

[ ]   [ ]   [ ]   Are chairs and other furniture in good condition?

[ ]   [ ]   [ ]   Are all compressed gas cylinders which may be in your area secured from falling over?

[ ]   [ ]   [ ]   During the survey, were all staff observed to use proper body mechanics?

[ ]   [ ]   [ ]   In areas where items are stored or placed overhead, is there ready access to a suitable stepstool, stepladder, or similar device?

[ ]   [ ]   [ ]   In storage areas, are the heavier items stored at waist level, with the lightest objects placed on the higher shelves?

[ ]   [ ]   [ ]   Is your area free of items which are likely to cause eye or head injuries, or which create an unusual bumping hazard? (Consider the use of protective padding.)

[ ]   [ ]   [ ]   Are all vehicles (cards, wheelchairs, etc.) in good operating condition?

Please list any comments made by staff in your area, or your own observations, which may help reduce accidents.

Electrical Safety

Date: _____   Location: _____

Surveyor: _____

YES NO N/A

[ ] [ ] [ ] Does all electrical equipment in patient care areas have a valid safety inspection decal. (N/A for battery-powered devices.)

[ ] [ ] [ ] Is access to electrical panels clear and not obstructed?

[ ] [ ] [ ] Are all electrical switches & circuit breakers identified?

   If not, list the locations of those which are not on the back of this sheet.

[ ] [ ] [ ] Are all electrical receptacles and cover plates in good condition?

[ ] [ ] [ ] Are electrical cords and plugs in good condition? Check for damaged insulation, cut cords, splices, and tape wrapped around the cord - none of which should be present.

[ ] [ ] [ ] Are extension cords in the area of the 3 wire (3-pins on the plug) type?

[ ] [ ] [ ] Have all extension cords been approved for use by Engineering?

[ ] [ ] [ ] Is the area completely free of electrical power cord adapters of any type, except where provided by the Engineering department?

[ ] [ ] [ ] Is all electrical equipment in the area visually in good condition?

[ ] [ ] [ ] Do personnel in the area know the hospital's policy & procedures for identifying and handling defective equipment?

1. Explain all NO items, or their locations, on this sheet. Be as specific as possible.
2. List the locations of ALL extension cords on this sheet.

Appendix G

Special Policy on Safety   Department of Radiology

Department of Radiology
Compliance with Guidelines for Safety

Policy: It is a paramount consideration in the operation of the
            Department that basic health and safety of the persons
            served and personnel are maintained in an appropriate
            manner. The Department will operate under the written
            plan of the Hospital for fire and other emergencies. And,
            the effectiveness of that plan will be tested on a regular
            basis. Comprehensive inspections of physical plant and
            adherence to all safety requirements that may be promul-
            gated by state, federal and local authorities will be con-
            ducted on a yearly basis and managed under the auspices
            of the Director of Plant Engineering.

General Safety Precautions

Needles, broken glass, and other sharps will be disposed of properly.

Drawers will be kept closed at all times when not actually in use.

Chairs and other furniture will be maintained and in good condition.

In areas where items are stored or placed overhead, there will be
ready access to a suitable stepstool, stepladder or similar device.

In storage areas, the heavier items will be stored at waist level, with
the lightest objects placed on the higher shelves.

The area will be free of items which are likely to cause eye or head
injuries, or which create an unusual bumping hazard.

All vehicles (carts, wheelchairs, etc.) will be maintained and in good
operating condition.

Refrigerators containing pharmaceuticals will be free of personal
food products and beverages.

All fire alarm boxes and fire extinguishers will be readily identifiable
and accessible.

All staff will know the locations of at least 2 fire extinguishers in, on,
or near their work area.

Staff in the area will be familiar with the location of the Disaster Manual and the Safety Manual.

Staff in the area will know the proper reporting procedure if they find (or believe there may be) a fire.

When Fire is Known or Suspected:

1. Remove persons from immediate danger.
2. Report the fire by first pulling down on the fire alarm (located next to each exit stairway).
3. Call the operator using the emergency number - 2222 and give the exact location of the fire.
4. Close all windows and doors.
5. Extinguish the fire ONLY after the above has been done.
6. Smoke must be reported as a fire. Strange odors which may be smoke or from fire may be either reported as a fire or just phoned into the hospital operator—but don't just let the situation go unreported. . . we must check out all possible fire situations.
7. Refer to BHET Fire Plan for further instructions.

Nothing will be stored closer than 18 inches from the ceiling.

All containers of powder, liquids and gases will be labeled to indicate what they contain.

NO SMOKING signs will be prominently posted wherever oxygen cylinders are present, oxygen flowmeters are plugged into the wall (whether in use or not) or oxygen is being administered.

All wastebaskets and ashtrays in the area will be of non-combustible material.

The area will be free of portable space heaters.

Any carts, wheelchairs, and/or other times in the corridors will be placed along the same side of the hall, or otherwise placed so that they do not create an obstacle course.

The corridors will be reasonably clear of obstructions.

Any wet floors will be marked with CAUTION, WET FLOOR (or similar) signs or reported to housekeeping.

The carpeting secure to the floor will be unfrayed, free from tripping hazards, and generally in good condition, or reported to Plant Engineering.

Hard floor surfaces will be secure to the floor and free of tripping and slipping hazards.

All EXIT signs will be illuminated or reported to Plant Engineering.

When opened and then released, all fire doors will close and latch properly or reported to Plant Engineering.

General Evacuation Plan:

1. Instructions for evacuation will be issued by Administration and the Department Director.
2. Evacuate stable patients with charts by bed or stretcher, if elevator operating; one staff member to each patient.
3. Evacuate patients by elevators.
4. If elevators are not operating, evacuate patients by stretcher down the nearest stairwell.
5. During evacuation, each section coordinator is responsible for knowing the whereabouts of each patient.

Body Mechanics/Back Care

All staff will observe proper body mechanics.

Staff will never attempt to lift or more any person, or object, unless they feel they can safely do so.

Staff will call for assistance when needed to move or lift patients.

Disaster Plan/Contingency Plan

All Department areas will participate in the hospital disaster and contingency plans as specified by those plans. Refer to those sections of the Emergency Preparedness Manual.

Hazardous Materials/Waste

The Department will participate in the hospital plan as specified in the Hazardous Communication Manual located in each area.

Infection Control

Each section within the Department will follow guidelines as specified in Infection Control procedures in each department's manual.

4.9 RISK MANAGEMENT AND LIABILITY PREVENTION

The current environment of professional liability and risk management in healthcare is one that faces providers with a clear responsibility to account to the public for the quality of its services. It's ironic that this increased accountability for the risks and uncertainties inherent to the provision of healthcare services comes at a point where modern medicine is better than ever. The alarmingly litigious nature of healthcare has led the Joint Commission on Accreditation of Healthcare Organizations to assume a leading role in the promotion of risk management activities. There are several references to risk management in the *Accreditation Manual For Hospitals, 1992.* In the Management and Administrative Services section of the manual, risk management and liability prevention activities are supported by the following standard:

- **MA 1.6** The chief executive officer, through the management and administrative staff, provides support for MA.1.6.1 the medical staff in the following activities:
  —MA.1.6.1.1 the identification of general areas of potential risk in the clinical aspects of patient care and safety;
  —MA.1.6.1.2 the development of criteria for identifying speciic cases with potential risk in the clinical aspects of patient care and safety and evaluation of these cases;
  —MA.1.6.1.3 the correction of problems in the clinical aspects of patient care and safety identified by risk management activities; and
  —MA.1.6.1.4 the design of programs to reduce risk in the clinical aspects of patient care and safety.

Risk management is the process of avoiding or controlling risk of financial loss to healthcare practitioners or institutions. Risk management is a matter of patient safety; it is obvious that poor quality care that creates a risk of injury to patients will lead to increased financial liability.

In many healthcare organizations, the risk management department and the quality assurance department are together and very often share a department head. The quality assurance function is intended to identify and resolve problems with patient care and to suggest opportunities to improve patient care. Risk management is engaged in the protection of financial assets by managing insurance for potential liability by reducing liability through surveillance. The practical similarities of these two management areas makes them good administrative roommates. Both aim to identify and resolve problems and both depend on established screening criteria and the timely flow of information needed to identify problems and to evaluate corrective actions.

Risk management, as it relates to patient care, will identify actual and potential causes of patient accidents and will implement programs to eliminate or reduce these occurrences. In 1983 the St. Paul Insurance Company published a summary of hospital malpractice claims by location in the hospital. The summary revealed that radiology services ranked in the top four services in claims activity.

The Legal Environment

No mention of the legal environment of healthcare today would be complete without discussing the landmark healthcare decision of *Darling v. Charleston Community Memorial Hospital* in 1965. This important case demonstrated society's changing attitude about the accountability for care rendered within a healthcare facility. In this particular case, the court ruled that the hospital was responsible for supervising the care of a patient in that hospital and their failure to properly monitor that patient's condition constituted a breach of the hospital's corporate responsibility. Before the Darling case decision, the allied health professional enjoyed the protection of legal theory that viewed the physician as the "captain of the ship." The theory that hospital employees are merely extensions of the physician in the care of the patient is not true. The courts decided that the hospital has a duty to protect its patients. Under the doctrine of respondeat superior, "let the master answer," a healthcare facility is held responsible for the actions of the allied health professionals who work there. This accountability for these healthcare professionals' actions stems from the organization's authority to regulate hiring, tenure, and work performed. Students of basic economics will recognize the doctrine of caveat emptor, "let the buyer beware." It expresses an old idea in common law that the buyer has a responsibility to protect himself from the seller. Modern healthcare has turned that doctrine around to the idea of caveat venditor, "let the seller beware."

The modern hospital owes five important duties to its patients:

- To exercise reasonable care in providing medical equipment, supplies, drugs and food.
- To exercise reasonable care in assuring a safe environment.
- Policies and procedures that will reasonably protect the safety of patients.
- To take reasonable care in the selection of hospital employees and to review continued clinical competence.
- To exercise reasonable care to guarantee that adequate care is provided.

Technological advances in imaging have increased the risk of equipment-related malpractice claims. Equipment-related malpractice claims usually are a result of:

- Failure to properly orient users that incorrect operation or misuse of equipment will cause serious injury.
- Failure to educate operators in the proper use of equipment.
- Failure to maintain records of periodic repair or inspection of equipment.

Each of these failures would be easy to prevent with a proper orientation program and inservice education to operators of the equipment. A comprehensive equipment quality control program that includes operator training will lessen equipment problems.

Before a malpractice suit is successful in obtaining a settlement for a client, there needs to be clearly documented violations in some standard areas:

- Standard of care must be compromised. It must be proved that an incident occurred as a result of some substandard behavior or procedure on the part of the caregiver.

- Breach of duty or violation of the standard of care must be committed. For instance, the wrong equipment might be used during a radiographic procedure, or the wrong procedure is performed.
- Proximate cause of the causal relation between the breach and the event causing injury must be proven. If a patient is hurt during an examination and the radiographer caused that hurt through carelessness, the radiographer is liable.
- Injury must occur.

Responding to Court Subpoenas

Healthcare providers are most often required to produce documents by court subpoena and on occasion will testify through deposition or trial. The majority of subpoenas are requests for medical records. They do not require the provider to be present or to testify in court. Most of the time, the original record must be sent and will be returned. Always make a copy of any record you submit to a legal proceeding. Never make alterations, deletions, or additions to any records that are subpoenaed to court. The subpoena is a document issued by the court calling for testimony at a given time, date, and location. The two types of discovery subpoenas most often received by healthcare providers are requests for records and requests for depositions (live testimony by witnesses).

A deposition subpoena results in a formal interview that will take place before a trial. Its purpose is to discover facts from a witness prior to the trial. At a deposition, one or more attorneys will ask questions about the qualifications of the witness and their knowledge of any facts pertinent to the case to be tried. Answers to questions are recorded by a court reporter who will prepare a transcript of the deposition. The witness has a right to request a copy of the transcript and take the opportunity to review it and make corrections.

Another type of subpoena is the deposition subpoena *duces tecum*, which requires that a witness bring documents to a deposition. Usually, these documents are in the possession of a particular department and that department head, who is custodian of the records, is the person who delivers those records to the place of the deposition. Never leave original records at a deposition; original materials should never be turned over to an attorney without a court order or a release from the patient. The costs of copying records is always borne by the requesting attorney.

A trial subpoena requires the witness' presence to testify before a judge or jury. In many cases the receipt of the trial subpoena will be the first notice of involvement that a provider will have in the case. A trial subpoena will always include the date and time of the trial. Trial dates change frequently; therefore, always check with the attorney who issued the subpoena and make arrangements to be notified of the actual trial date.

Careful preparation is necessary prior to giving testimony. Always review any records you have carefully prior to the testimony at a trial. Also, if you have been a witness at a deposition, review the testimony at the deposition as well in order to avoid any inconsistencies in your testimony.

Never ignore a subpoena. The attorney who issued the subpoena can initiate contempt proceedings, which are very expensive to defend. Additionally, a judge presiding over a case can order you to appear at an arbitrary time, actually send a sheriff to bring you to court, and charge you for court costs.

Reducing Patient Anxiety Will Avoid Trouble Later

From the patient's standpoint, the most intimidating aspect of the imaging procedure is coping with the anxiety associated with it. Consider the mental status of the patient who receives radiographs ordered to rule out cancer. The patient is in a state of high anxiety over the possibility that some terrible tumor might be found. The patient worries that something will go wrong during the procedure, that the results of the procedure may be interpreted incorrectly, or that he may receive the wrong procedure. When preparing patients for procedures in the radiology department, the radiologist and the radiographer should pay close attention to the patient's readiness for the procedure. Failure to establish and maintain rapport with the patient is the root of most complaints that lead to malpractice cases. Patients do not expect to be cured of every medical problem, but they do expect to be treated courteously and with some sympathy. When a patient encounters an indifferent and aloof caretaker, they react with anger. Extensive research has documented that patients who are adequately prepared and reassured about the procedure that they are about to undergo will experience less pain and fewer complications. When preparing a patient for an invasive radiological procedure, the following steps are helpful in alleviating patient anxiety:

- Establish good rapport with the patient. Call the patient by name, be sympathetic, and maintain good eye contact.
- Tell the patient about the procedure and describe the sensations the patient may experience; use an instructional brochure to reenforce important information about the procedure.
- Encourage the patient to relax; common effective relaxation techniques include deep breathing, distraction, and imagery. Try to gauge the patient's emotional status by asking the patient how he feels. Talk about anxiety and the reasons for that anxiety.
- Stay with the patient during the procedure and offer encouragement and reassurance.

A Liability Prevention Checklist for the Radiology Manager

By John C. Lenahan, Esquire
Evenson, Wand, Edwards, Lenahan & McKeown
1200 G. Street N.W., Suite 700
Washington, D.C. 20005

1. Competence.
    a. Review the certification and qualifications of the radiologic technologists.
    b. Encourage the technologists to continue their education and to participate in professional associations and activities.
    c. Keep a record of any continuing education courses attended by the technologists.
    d. Maintain an accessible library of current professional literature.
    e. Conduct in-service training.

2. Compliance.
   a. Establish policies and procedures for the Radiology Department.
   b. Publish the procedures and ensure by written acknowledgement and certification of the technologists that they have read and familiarized themselves with the policies and procedures.
   c. Review the policies and procedures, adopt new ones, and modify or delete old ones.
   d. Personally monitor compliance with procedures from time-to-time and counsel technologists regarding the purpose and benefits of compliance.
3. Charting.
   a. Remind the staff that the chart is a legal document and of its importance in terms of healthcare and potential lawsuits.
   b. Emphasize to the staff the importance of accurate and prompt reporting to the patient's charts.
4. Communication.
   a. Ensure open lines of communication between your department and others in the hospital.
   b. Ensure communication within the department, including a suggestion box and periodic staff meetings, and maintain a file of bulletins and memoranda concerning the policies, procedures, and practices of the department.
   c. Emphasize the importance of appropriate verbal and nonverbal communication skills on the part of the technologist, including a neat x-ray room, neat personal appearance, and a courteous manner in dealing with the patients, patients' family members, and other members of the hospital staff.
   d. Establish and review procedures for communication with nonEnglish speaking patients and patients with other disabilities who are unable to communicate in the normal verbal manner.
5. Confidentiality.
   a. Ensure that the staff understands and maintains the confidentiality of patients' identities and records, including x-rays.

b. Ensure that no information on a patient is released to anyone not entitled to know without a properly signed release or medical authorization, or a court subpoena.

c. Consult with the hospital's in-house risk manager or legal counsel for the answer to questions concerning the release of information.

6. Courtesy.

a. Establish a policy and emphasize to the staff the need to be courteous in dealing with patients, patients' family members, and other members of the staff, and to treat all patients with equal dignity and respect, emphasizing the importance of such treatment not only in regard to good quality care but also in the prevention of lawsuits.

7. Carefulness.

a. Review the adequacy and state of the art of the equipment.

b. Ensure regular preventative maintenance is being performed.

c. Ensure that high quality film is being used.

d. Publish periodic safety bulletins emphasizing the importance of safety generally and specific areas of potential risk particularly.

e. Ensure that proper patient identification techniques are being used, methods for preventing patient falls are known, adequate x-ray files are maintained, and other areas of safety concern are reviewed, to ensure that patient care is managed safely and without incident.

Informed Consent

A most critical and controversial issue in healthcare today is the doctrine of informed consent. The issue of consent is not new. Based in common law, the concept of personal autonomy and self-determination was upheld in the Illinois Courts with the case of *Pratt v. Davis*, 1905.

The doctrine of informed consent is that before a patient undergoes any procedure, he must be told about the procedure, the risks of death or bodily harm inherent with the procedure, the benefits of the procedure, the alternatives and their consequences, and the expectations about recuperation. An exception to this rule occurs when a patient has an emergent risk to life and the law allows consent to a physician to perform procedures to protect the patient's well-being.

The concept of informed consent is a special form of communication between provider and patient. It assumes:

1. Patients do not understand medical science.
2. An adult of sound mind has the right to refuse medical treatment.
3. Consent, to be valid, must be informed.
4. The patient must rely on his physician for the information necessary to make the decision to submit to treatment.

Informed medical consent is an important medical legal question that raises legal, ethical, and practical issues for radiologic practitioners. Because of the procedure-oriented nature of radiology as a specialty, radiologists must obtain informed consent from their patients almost daily. Informed consent usually grows naturally out of the normal physician-patient relationship. Over time, a rapport builds that allows the management of informed consent to be a natural action. Unfortunately, in the case of patient-radiologist relationships, contact is brief and episodic. Therefore, many radiologists view the procedure of informed consent with some discomfort and consider obtaining that consent to be a legal imposition. Instead, the informed consent procedure should be approached as an avenue to assure an adequately informed patient as a defense against a malpractice suit. It is also the time to learn about the patient and give that patient an opportunity to gather confidence in the radiologist performing the procedure.

Informed Consent in Radiology

The wider use of informed consent procedures in radiology is primarily due to the continued incidence of serious and fatal reactions to iodinated contrast media. There are 10 million contrast-enhanced radiological examinations performed in the United States every year. Even with the use of new nonionic contrast agents, the risk of adverse reactions is still significant. Contrast reaction lawsuits make up the greater part of radiology-related losses to malpractice carriers. The broader use of informed consent procedures in radiology is encouraged by risk managers, insurance carriers, and hospital attorneys.

From a practical standpoint, a limited number of procedures in radiology require informed consent. Most of these procedures involve the IV injection of contrast material.   At the very least, patients having contrast-enchanced exams should be informed of six elements relating to the procedure to be performed:

1. The diagnosis and condition of the patient.
2. The purpose of the examination.
3. The risks generally associated with the examination.
4. The expected success of the examination.
5. Alternatives to the examination.
6. Prognosis without the examination.

A successful litigation can be avoided if none of the four causes of action described here can be demonstrated by the plaintiff.

1. The physician must inform the patient of serious risks.
2. The physician must give the patient enough information to make an informed decision to accept or reject the examination.
3. The patient would have declined the procedure if the risks of contrast agent use were fully understood.
4. An injury occurred as a result of the examination.

A written informed consent procedure (see Figure 4.17) is the best defense for a malpractice suit concerning consent. Malpractice becomes difficult to prove when patients are informed of benefits, risks, and alternatives to IV contrast medias and when that informed consent is signed by the patient. An additional safeguard is to chart in the patient's medical record that an informed consent discussion took place.

Figure 4.17 Special Consent to Operation or Other Procedure

Patient_____ Date_____ Time _____ (a.m./p.m.)
1. I hereby authorize Dr._____ and/or such assistants as may be selected by him, and the medical staff at the _____ Hospital, to remedy the condition or conditions which appear indicated by the diagnostic studies already performed. _____
   (Explain the nature of the condition and the need to remedy such condition)
2. The procedure(s) necessary to be performed (has, have) been explained to me by Dr. _____ and I understand the nature of the procedure to be:
   _____
   (A description of procedure in laymen's terms)
3. Procedure as scheduled: _____
4. It has been explained to me that, during the course of the operation, unforeseen condition(s) may be revealed that necessitate(s) an extension of the original procedure(s) or different procedure(s) than those set forth in Paragraph 2. I therefore authorize and request that the above named physician, his assistants, or his designees perform such medical and surgical procedures as are necessary and desirable in the exercise of professional judgment. The authority granted under this Paragraph 3 shall extend to remedying all conditions that require treatment and are not known to Dr. _____ or the medical staff of the _____ Hospital at the time the operation is commenced.
5. I have been advised of risks and consequences associated with these procedures and also of other risks such as loss of blood, infection, and cardiac arrest which are attendant on the performance of any surgical or medical procedure. I am further aware that the practice of medicine and surgery is not an exact science and acknowledge that no guarantees have been made to me concerning the risks of this operation or procedure.
6. I consent to the administration of anesthesia to be applied by a qualified member of the anesthesia staff approved by my physician/ surgeon and the _____ Hospital, and to the use of such anesthetics as may be deemed advisable, with the exception of _____
7. I consent to the taking and publication of any photographs in the course of this operation for the purpose of advancing medical education.
8. I hereby give permission for the use of tissues removed to be used for scientific and experimental purposes as may be deemed appropriate by my attending physician or other person authorized by representatives of _____ Hospital.
9. I CERTIFY THAT I HAVE READ AND FULLY UNDERSTAND THE ABOVE INFORMATION. INAPPLICABLE PARAGRAPHS WERE STRICKEN BEFORE I SIGNED.

_____
(Signature)
(If patient is unable to sign or is a minor, complete the following): Patient (is a minor __ years of age) is unable to sign because: _____
_____

_____   _____
(Witness)   (Closest Relative or Legal Guardian)

                                      _____
                                      (Relationship)

Obtaining Consent

The physician is the one who must explain the risks, benefits, and alternatives of a procedure to the patient. Under ordinary rules of law, the physician may delegate the process of obtaining consent to an agent. That agent may be another physician, nurse, or technologist. The radiologist, as the principal physician performing the procedure, is still ultimately responsible and is liable for any mistakes in procedure that his agent makes while obtaining consent.

Criteria for the Use of Nonionic Contrast Media

In 1989, the Committee on Drugs and Contrast Media of the American College of Radiology (ACR) concluded that nonionic contrast media is safer to use than ionic agents. They based this finding on the results of two extensive studies involving more than one half million participants. Those studies reported that the incidence of severe reactions to ionic media was six times greater than with nonionic media. The studies further revealed that known high risk patients with allergies, asthma, and cardiovascular disease experienced fewer reactions with the administration of nonionic media as compared to low risk patients receiving conventional ionic agents. The conclusion drawn is that the major risk factor for a severe reaction to a contrast agent is not the presence of known risk factors, but the type of contrast used.

Implications for Use

The decision to switch to any new medical advance must be supported with the evidence that a greater degree of medical benefit exists. Nonionic medias cost about ten times more than ionics. In this environment of cost-containment and prospective payment, the economic aspect of this nonionic versus ionic debate is the contributing factor responsible for the relatively slow integration of this medical advance into standard radiological practice. From the administrative viewpoint, choosing ionics over nonionics strictly on the basis of cost is becoming increasingly unsupportable. Economic reasons that pressure clinical decision making are not easy to defend from the legal standpoint nor from an ethical one. If litigation results from a severe reaction or death following the administration of an ionic media to a known high risk patient, an argument based on economics will not stand up well against the six times safer record of the nonionic experience. On the other hand, a community standard of care defense is still a plausible argument because two types of contrast media are currently in use with no consensus standard existing. The community standard of care defense, however, becomes weaker as the conversion to nonionics gains momentum following the increased evidence of their safety.

Managing the Risk

There is a strong need for a decision-making framework using patient safety and clinical risk factors to assure the highest standards of care. Financial restraints will continue to necessitate the choice between the two types of contrast media. See figure 4.18 for standard quidelines.

Strict criteria should be used to determine which patients receive each contrast type. (See Figure 4.19) Detailed informed consent procedures need to be in place, including an explanation to the patient about contrast media choices. The controversy over the extent to which nonionic medias will replace older ionic agents for intravascular use in diagnostic studies is complicated by the multifactors of patient safety, comfort, standard of care, legal issues, economics, and reimbursement. In modern radiological practice, an awareness of the consequences surrounding the choice of contrast is just another necessary evil of doing business.

Figure 4.18   Guide to the use of non-ionic contrast media

Standard guidelines
Although many types of protocols are used throughout the country, the basic protocol for administering non-ionics usually consists of the following six criteria:

- patients who have experienced a previous contrast reaction
- coronary patients
- diabetics
- very ill patients
- elderly patients
- very young patients

Figure 4.18 (Continued)

While protocols vary with each hospital, the rationale is consistent in that non-ionics are used whenever above-average risk is present.

Some hospitals have elected to use non-ionics or low osmolality contrast on all patients due to the feelings of some physicians who dislike the idea of differentiating patients for contrast application.

In some cases, the referring physicians were given the option of selecting the contrast for their patients; however, this practice was found to be impractical and generally unacceptable.

Patient's choice

At one hospital, the radiologist decided to let each patient decide which types of contrast to use. This process works as follows:

1.   A form outlining the basic differences in the two types of contrast is given to each patient who is a candidate for an examination in which a contrast media is indicated.

The form is written in very basic language, using terminology that the average patient can understand.

The safety factor is emphasized and the relative cost of the two contrast types is pointed out.

2.   If the patient is unable to read or comprehend the information, a technologist assists him or her. Once the form has been read or explained, the patient signs what is now considered a consent form.

3.   In cases in which the patient decides to have the ionic contrast and has a history of contrast reactions or coronary disease, or if other high-risk factors are present, the technologist notifies the radiologist. In turn, the radiologist speaks to the patient in an attempt to clarify the benefits of using the non-ionic.*

Figure 4.19 Report of the Current Criteria for the Use of Water Soluble Contrast Agents for Intravenous Injections from the American College of Radiology's Committee on Drugs and Contrast Media

Section I. Introduction

The Committee on Drugs and Contrast Media of the Commission on Education of the American College of Radiology was given the charge to advise the members of the American College of Radiology regarding the appropriate use of contrast agents. In undertaking this task, the committee's objective was to review thoroughly and in detail the scientific evidence to date.

Recommendations have been formulated to provide as much protection as possible to individual patients receiving intravenous contrast media, while at the same time being cognizant of the importance of the economic issues and the potential for efficacious alternative uses of healthcare dollars. The previous report of this committee represents the committee's recommendations based on the scientific evidence through May 1988.

This report represents the committee's view based on scientific evidence available since that time. It must be recognized that the conclusions reached in this report are subject to revision as more evidence becomes available.

---

*Hunton, B.W. Protocols: Guide use of non-ionic contrast media. Advance for Administrators. 2(5):11, 1992.

Figure 4.19   (continued)

Section II.   General Considerations
There is now more scientific information available regarding the incidence of adverse reactions from the use of contrast agents.   The committee wishes to reemphasize some general principles:

1. Regardless of the clinical site, appropriately trained medical personnel, emergency medical equipment and medication should be readily available to treat any adverse reaction that might occur.
2. All patients referred for contrast examinations should be appropriately screened for the presence of risk factors that might increase the likelihood of adverse reactions.
3. All patients undergoing a contrast study should be adequately prepared prior to the examination, including adequate hydration and appropriate premedication when indicated.
4. If significant risk factors are present, it is prudent to seriously consider alternative diagnostic procedures that could provide the necessary information without using iodinated water soluble contrast agents.
5. The American College of Radiology recognizes the appropriateness of the use of any approved contrast agent, in accordance with the radiologist's best judgment.

When the decision is made to perform a contrast examination, the individual radiologist taking care of a specific patient must make a decision regarding the use of either higher osmolality contrast agents (HOCA) or lower osmolality contrast agents (LOCA). It cannot be over emphasized that each patient undergoing each type of contrast examination requires a consideration of the specific situation. In the final analysis, the radiologist (in consultation with the referring physician when necessary) is responsible for that patient and the radiological examination the patient is to undergo, and the radiologist is in the best position to design the study, properly prepare the patient as indicated by the specific clinical circumstances, and select the appropriate contrast material.

Section III.   Higher Osmolality Contrast Agents (HOCA)
HOCA for intravenous injections have been utilized in radiological examinations for approximately 60 years. Since first introduced, there has been progressive improvement in the quality of these agents in terms of usefulness of contrast material and safety. They are regarded by the medical community (including radiology) and the Food and Drug Administration as safe and effective. However, there is evidence suggesting that pretreatment with steroids (a two-dose steroid pretreatment regimen) before administering HOCA may further decrease patient risk. Subsequent reports may clarify the usefulness of steroids.

Nevertheless, because of the discomfort associated with the use of HOCA and the uncommon severe adverse reactions, the search for improved contrast agents continued. This resulted in the development of lower osmolality contrast agents, most of which are nonionic compounds.

Section IV.   Lower Osmolality Contrast Agents (LOCA)*
The nonionic agents have been shown to be associated with less discomfort and have a lower incidence of severe adverse reactions.

---

*Data concerning intravenous use of the ionic dimer (ioxaglate) are insufficient for these proposed guidelines.

Reprinted with the permission of the American College of Radiology from the *ACR Bulletin* 10/90.

Figure 4.19   (continued)

Some radiological facilities have decided to use lower osmolality contrast agents on all patients.

Other radiological facilities have decided on the selective use of LOCA. In these institutions, radiologists should give specific consideration to the use of LOCA and utilize the following guidelines that are based on the currently available evidence:

1. Patients with a history of a previous adverse reaction to contrast material, with the exception of a sensation of heat, flushing, or a single episode of nausea or vomiting.
2. Patients with a history of asthma or allergy.
3. Patients with known cardiac dysfunction, including recent or potentially imminent cardiac decompensation, severe arrhythmias, unstable angina pectoris, recent myocardial infarction, and pulmonary hypertension.
4. Patients with generalized severe debilitation.
5. Any other circumstances where, after due consideration, the radiologist believes there is a specific indication for the use of LOCA.

Examples of this include, but are not restricted to:

a. Sickle cell disease.
b. Patients at increased risk for aspiration.
c. Patients who are manifestly very anxious about the contrast procedure.
d. Patients with whom communication cannot be established in order to determine the presence or absence of risk factors.
e. Patients who request or demand the use of LOCA.

Appendix A—Do's and Don'ts of Malpractice Risk Management*

- Do communicate abnormal results uncovered in the final reading of images ordered from the emergency room. The risk of litigation increases when there is no clear line of communication between the radiologist and the patient's physician. For example, the patient may mistakenly believe his condition is normal and he may not have a personal physician to inform him otherwise. It is then the radiologist's responsibility to make sure the hospital finds the patient to disclose the new findings.
- Don't falsify or destroy evidence. This is the surest way to lose a malpractice suit. Wrongdoing is almost always uncovered and will be used against you.
- Do deal with erroneous patient expectations. Communication protocols should be in place to inform patients about the differences

*Brice, J. "Simple Tactics Minimize Exposure to Malpractice." *Diagnostic Imaging*. 14(3):44-5, 1992.

between a consulting physician and an attending physician and how that distinction applies to this medical encounter.

- Don't administer ionic contrast or perform an invasive procedure without informed consent. Emergencies justify violating this rule. If it is a routine procedure and the patient does not speak English, delay the study until you administer the informed consent through a translator.
- Do understand and follow ACR guidelines. Because radiologists are judged on a national standard of care, the American College of Radiology guidelines are certain to be used as evidence in court.

The new ACR communication guidelines are particularly important. Radiologists should comply with recommendations on when they should personally phone referring physicians. These include: when the diagnosis necessitates immediate case management decisions; when potentially life-threatening diagnoses are detected; when emergency or primary reports conflict with the final report; and when potentially significant, incidental findings are made during other studies.

- Don't delegate informed consent to others. You can't testify whether documentation describing informed consent was accurate if you weren't there to witness it.
- Do document the medical record when departing from standards of care. ACR guidelines do not cover every contingency, so radiologists are free to proceed with actions that deviate from the college's recommendations. The rationale for noncompliance, however, should be clearly documented in the medical record.
- Do compile legible and complete medical records. The medical record almost always works in the radiologist's favor in court, so it is important that text is readable and well-organized. One should use good penmanship in blue or black ink (never pencil). All entries should be dated and initialed. Tape transcriptions should be proofread. When making changes, draw a single line through the entry, then initial and date the addendum.
- Do record curbstone consults. The standards of accountability do not diminish when the radiologist informally volunteers advice. Keep a diary documenting those consultations as accurate records that describe exactly what was said.
- Don't talk to plaintiff's counsel before contacting your malpractice insurer and its attorney. You need professional help the instant the plaintiff's attorney makes the call.

- Do always include the following language in your informed consent and in the medical record documenting it: "The benefits, alternatives, and risks—including death, organ damage and paralysis—have been discussed with the patient, who acknowledges and accepts them." This documentation can serve as your ironclad defense.
- Don't incriminate yourself when facing a legal challenge. In a potential lawsuit, never review the film evidence with your colleagues. The content of those meetings will be used as evidence against you.

Appendix B*

The Council of the American College of Radiology adopted Resolution 5, a standard for communication, at the 1991 Council meeting. The text of that standard follows:

ACR Standard for Communication—Diagnostic Radiology

Communication is a critical component of the art and science of medicine and is especially important in diagnostic radiology. Diagnostic radiology is one of the most important consultative services in medicine.

The final product of any consultation is the submission of a report on the results of the consultation. In addition, the diagnostic radiologist and the referring physician have many opportunities to communicate directly with each other during the course of a patient's case management. Such communication should be encouraged because it leads to more effective and appropriate utilization of diagnostic radiology in addressing clinical problems and focuses attention on such concerns as radiation exposure, appropriate imaging studies, clinical efficacy, and cost-effective examinations.

In order to afford optimal care to the patient and enhance the cost effectiveness of each diagnostic examination, radiological consultations ought to be provided and radiographs interpreted within a known clinical setting. The ACR supports radiologists who insist on clinical data with each consultation request.

---

*Used with the permission of the Council of the ACR and reprinted from the *ACR Bulletin* 11/91.

A. The Diagnostic Radiology Report

An authenticated written interpretation should be performed on all radiologic (imaging) procedures. The report should include the following items:

1. Name of patient and another identifier, such as birthdate, Social Security number, or hospital or office identification number.
2. Name of the referring physician.
   Rationale: To provide more accurate routing of the report to one or more locations specified by the referring physician (hospital, office, clinic, etc.). Each department should develop a policy to insure proper distribution of the written report to the hospital chart and referring (attending) physician for all inpatients and the referring physician for all outpatients.
3. Name or type of examination.
4. Dates of the examination and transcription.
   Rationale: To permit tracking of the report.
5. Time of the examination (for ICU-CCU patients).
   Rationale: To identify multiple examinations (e.g. chest) that may be performed on a single day.
6. Body of the report.
   a. *Procedures and Materials*
      Include in the report a description of the procedures performed and any contrast media (agent, concentration, volume and reaction, if any), medications, catheters, and devices, if not reported elsewhere.
      Rationale: To ensure accurate communication and be available for future reference.
   b. *Findings*
      Use precise anatomical and radiological terminology to describe the findings accurately.
   c. *Limitations*
      Where appropriate, identify factors that can limit the sensitivity and specificity of the examination.
      Comment: Such factors might include technical factors, patient anatomy (e.g., dense breast pattern), limitations of the technique (e.g., chest examination for pulmonary embolism), incomplete bowel preparation (e.g., barium enema for neoplasm), wrist examination for carpal scaphoid injury, or skeletal examination for detection of stress fracture.

The standards of the American College of Radiology (ACR) are not rules but attempt to define principles of practice which should generally produce high quality radiological care. The radiologist may exceed an existing standard as determined by the individual patient and available resources. The standards should not be deemed inclusive of all proper methods of care or exclusive of other methods of care reasonably directed to obtaining the same results. The ultimate judgment regarding the propriety of any specific procedure or course of conduct must be made by the radiologist in light of all circumstances presented by the individual situation. Adherence to ACR standards will not assure successful outcome in every situation. It is prudent to document the rationale for any deviation from these suggested standards in the radiologist's policies and procedures manual or, if not addressed there, in the patient's medical record.

    d. *Clinical Issues*

       The report should address or answer any pertinent clinical issues raised in the request for the imaging examination. *Comment:* For example, to rule out pneumothorax, state "There is no evidence of pneumothorax," or to rule out fracture, "There is no evidence of fracture." It is not advisable to use such universal disclaimers as "The mammography examination does not exclude the possibility of cancer."

    e. *Comparative Data*

       Comparisons with previous examinations and reports when possible are a part of the radiologic consultation and report and optionally may be part of the "impression" section.

7. Impression (Conclusion or Diagnosis).

    a. Each examination should contain an "impression" section unless the study is being compared with other recent studies and no changes have occurred during the interval, or the body of the report is brief.

    b. Give a precise diagnosis whenever possible.

    c. Give a differential diagnosis when appropriate.

    d. Recommend, only when appropriate, follow-up and additional diagnostic radiologic studies to clarify or confirm the impression.

B. Written Communication

1. The timeliness of reporting any radiologic examination varies with the nature and urgency of the clinical problem. The written radiological report should be made available in a clinically

radiologcal report should be made available in a clinically appropriate, timely manner.

2. The final report should he proofread carefully to avoid typographical errors, deleted words, and confusing or conflicting statements, and signed (authenticated) by a radiologist, whenever possible.
   Comment: Electronic or rubber-stamp signature devices, instead of a written signature, are acceptable if access to them is secure. The signature of the radiologist who dictated the report should appear on the report. If this is not possible, the initials or name of the radiologist who dictated the report as well as the initials or name of the radiologist who signed it should appear on the report.

3. A copy of the final report should accompany the exchange of relevant radiographic examinations from one health professional to another health professional.

C. Direct Communication

1. Radiologists should attempt to coordinate their efforts with those of the referring physician in order to best serve the patient's well being. In some circumstances, such coordination may require direct communication of unusual, unexpected, or urgent findings to the referring physician in advance of the formal written report. Examples include:

   a. The probable detection of conditions carrying the risk of acute morbidity and/or mortality which may require immediate case management decisions.

   b. The probable detection of disease with non-acute morbidity or mortality sufficiently serious that it may require prompt notification of the patient, clinical evaluation or initiation of treatment.

2. In these circumstances, the radiologist, or his or her representative, should attempt to communicate directly (in person or by telephone) with the referring physician, or his or her representative. The timeliness of direct communication should be based upon the immediacy of the clinical situation.

3. Documentation of actual or attempted direct communication is appropriate in accordance with department policy, legal

advisability, understanding with the referring physician, and individual judgement.
4. Any discrepancy between an emergency or preliminary report and the final written report should be promptly reconciled by direct communication to the referring physician, or his or her representative.

Note: This standard is structured with statements of principles followed by rationales or comments. Only the principles define the range of suggested practices. The rationales or comments serve only to clarify the principles.

4.10 BASIC HEALTHCARE FINANCIAL MANAGEMENT

If you work in a large hospital, the same scene is played over and over again at department head meetings when the financial condition of your hospital is discussed by the chief financial officer. The present preoccupation is reducing days in accounts receivable and reducing length of stay. These are huge financial challenges that we face in managing hospitals in the era of prospective payment. In a greatly over simplified view of how modern hospitals run, the financial side of the organization is busy shaving days off of accounts receivable by dropping the bill faster, and the operations people are busy shaving days off of length of stay by dropping the patient out of the hospital faster. In a word, it would seem that as providers we are in a race to do it quicker and cheaper, with higher quality and customer satisfaction.

Many radiology managers today are responsible for huge operations budgets and manage the acquisition of millions of dollars of high technology equipment. How much does the average radiology manager need to know about healthcare finance? This chapter will attempt to introduce the subject of basic healthcare finance to the reader who needs to understand enough about hospital accounting procedures to function effectively in the radiology manager's role.

Voluntary Not-for-Profit Hospitals

Most hospitals in the United States are voluntary not-for-profit hospitals. They were originally organized by community residents for the benefit of the community, and the hospital is sustained solely for the purpose of public interest. These hospitals are organized as "not-for-profit," and this terminology means that no single individual or group of individuals directly benefits from the profits that might be derived from the operation of the hospital. In fact, by this definition any profits realized must be reinvested in the hospital for the purpose of expansion, renovation, or technological improvement. The term "not-for-profit" does not mean that the hospital is not trying to make money. Few organizations would survive in the long run without generating excess revenues. These excess revenues are required in an industry like healthcare to keep pace with inflation and the increasing demands of technology for patient care.

Where Revenue Comes From

Patients in our hospitals are classified according to the responsibility for the payment of their bills. The major classifications of payors are briefly described here.

On July 1, 1966, the national **Medicare** program became effective. The program was established to meet the healthcare needs of the elderly and disabled. Medicare is part of the Social Security Amendments of 1965 (Title XVIII), and these Medicare benefits are provided under two separate but closely related programs. Part A of Medicare provides payment for hospital services; Part B, which is also known as Supplementary Medical Insurance, provides professional payments to doctors and to many diagnostic services. Medicare coverage automatically accrues to social security beneficiaries who have reached the age of 65; Medicare Part B is a voluntary program that may be purchased at a nominal cost. Payment for services provided to Medicare patients is made directly to the hospital under Part A. The basis for payment to hospitals used to be reasonable costs of providing the services. Mature hospital managers will often refer to those cost-based times of reimbursement as "the good old days."

Prior to 1983, retrospective cost-based reimbursement was the main third-party payment mechanism. In that era, it encompassed not only capital costs, but also almost all other types of costs as well. In late 1983, Medicare phased out retrospective cost-based reimbursement in favor of the prospective payment system. Regulated rates were established for each of several hundred diagnostic related groups (DRGs) and other payors are rapidly following suite.

The primary goal of **Medicaid** is to provide for healthcare services to the indigent. Unlike Medicare, which is available to any social security recipient, benefits under Medicaid are only available to those defined by state law as needy, and Medicaid participation is not limited to any age group. Medicaid programs are administered at the state level and Medicaid programs differ from state to state. The costs of state Medicaid programs are shared by the individual states and the federal government. Reimbursement to hospitals for services provided to Medicaid recipients also differs from state to state. Most states have Medicaid programs with severe financial constraints.

Blue Cross is a nongovernment insurance program that covers healthcare services according to the terms of contracts that are individually negotiated as health plans for major employers. Reimbursement for healthcare services by Blue Cross plans can a be large percentage of hospital revenues. **Self-pay, commercial,** and **managed care** make up the remainder of the payors for healthcare. With commercial payors, reimbursement may be made directly to the patient or may be assigned to the hospital. With these categories of payors, the patient is ultimately responsible for the bill. Commercial insurance pays for healthcare services on a customary charge basis less whatever deductible arrangements may exist. Managed care payors negotiate discounts with providers and pay for healthcare services based on very specific plan provisions. Patients in a self-pay category pay their own hospital bill. Very few patients fall into the self-pay category.

Most of the hospital's total revenues will be derived from Medicare and commercial payors. In other industries, revenues generated from the sale of goods will equal the quantity of goods sold × the price per unit. This fundamental principle of accounting does not hold for hospitals. For the most part, a hospital is compensated on the basis of the defined cost of providing services rather than on list prices. The revenue generated by the services or procedures rendered to a patient will never equal the units sold × the price. This is why the term **contractual adjustment/allowance** is so important to healthcare accounting. Hospitals account for third-party payments as though they received full charges for services rendered. The difference between the list price of the service and the actual payment received by a third-party payor is called the "contractual adjustment" or "allowance." It is shown as a deduction from gross revenues in the financial statements of the organization.

Communicating Through Codes

When attempting to understand the complexities of healthcare reimbursement, a thorough understanding of how codes originated and are used will assist you in maximizing reimbursement. Ongoing changes due to government regulations will make coding a constant challenge to the radiology manager. (See Figure 4.20)

Diagnostic Coding—ICD–9–CM International Classification of Diseases, 9th Edition, Clinical Modification

The accuracy of coding cannot be emphasized enough. Coding must be performed correctly and consistently to provide meaningful statistics to aid in planning for health needs and health care. Transforming verbal descriptions of disease, injuries, conditions, and procedures into numerical designations (coding) is a complex activity and should not be undertaken without proper training.

If you have any questions regarding the use and interpretation of the ICD-9-CM text, you may contact: World Health Organization Center for Classification of Disease in North America, National Center for Health Statistics, Department of Health and Human Services, 3700 East-West Highway, Hyattsville, Maryland 20782.

Currently, there are three ICD-9-CM volumes designed for the classification of morbidity and mortality statistics.

Base Code

In coding ICD-9 the base term relates to a specific disease or disorder using three digits. A maximum of five digits are used in coding ICD-9. For example:

474	Chronic disease of tonsils and adenoids
474.1	Hypertrophy of tonsils and adenoids
474.10	Tonsils and adenoids

Figure 4.20   Reimbursement Lingo

Coding is the process of assigning numbers to healthcare terms. Because it creates standardized terminology, it is a vehicle for communication that is compatible with computerized operations. It is done in order to group conditions and procedures that are similar for multiple purposes—to create statistical tabulations, to determine patterns of diseases and services provided, to forecast and focus healthcare resources, to study epidemiology, to standardize reporting, to evaluate the quality of healthcare by outcomes, and to determine reimbursement policy and calculations.

CPT = Current Procedural Terminology. CPTs were developed by the AMA and are revised annually. The codes equate to descriptions of *procedures* that are used for reporting medical *services.* Each code consists of five digits. Most radiology procedures are included in 70000-79999.

HCPC = Medicare's Common Procedural Coding System. These may be substituted, if more accurate, or used to expand the CPT coding system to report *services* to Medicare. Most are alpha-numeric. National codes begin with the letters A-V; local offices may develop codes beginning with W-Z. Radiology services will begin with R followed by four digits. To date, very few are available. Medical and surgical supplies begin with A. By April 1990, A4648 is to be available for billing non-ionics, assuming the Medicare offices complete the computer system change required.

ICD9-CM = International Classification of Diseases Clinical Modifications ICD9-CM was developed by the World Health Organization. This system is revised every ten years to add new diagnoses. The primary purpose of this system is to classify diseases and etiologies into statistics for predicting trends and focusing healthcare resources. Medicare reviews ICD9s from claim data to evaluate and relate outcomes to the cost of care.

The ICD9 format is XXX.XX—three digits giving the base term (occasionally a letter and two digits), followed by a fourth and fifth digit that give detail and sub-categories. For example, 250.11 is the code for Diabetes. Ketoacidosis/Juvenile type; the 250 is for diabetes mellitus, the .1 for ketoacidosis, and the .01 for juvenile onset, in contrast to .00 for adult onset.

DRGs = Diagnostically Related Groupings DRGs are numerical codes, each designating a broad grouping of *diseases* primarily by body systems. A single payment level is attached to each and relates to reimbursement for inpatient hospital stays no matter what extent of care is provided. Variables considered in DRG assignment are the principal diagnosis, the principal operating room procedure, other diagnoses and procedures, the patient's age at admission, the patient's sex, and the discharge status. DRG levels can be increased by complicating (co-morbidity) diagnoses, particularly when more than one body system is affected.

Revenue Codes These three-digit codes may be used by hospitals for billing of inpatient or outpatient *services. Procedures* would require a corresponding CPT or HCPC code; *supplies* may not require this. The primary purpose of revenue codes is to identify and direct revenue and expenses to departments for accounting purposes.

RVS = Relative Value System The ACR and HCFA determined this system to equate units of service to a fee/payment schedule. The units are supposed to place a value based on the costs to provide a service including the skill level required, materials consumed, and time involved. Beginning October 1989, geographic factors are used as a multiplier when the RVS is used as the payment system for radiology clinics.

Dickes, Linda. *Reimbursement Lingo* from "Influencing Reimbursement." *RT Image.* July 16, 1990, p.17.

474.11   Tonsils alone
474.12   Adenoids alone

V Code

In supplemental classifications, the V Code should be used as primary diagnosis and used to code a patient's special health status. A maximum of five digits are used in coding the V Code. For example:

V10   Personal history of malignant neoplasm
V10.0   Gastrointestinal tract
V10.04   Stomach

E Codes

E Codes describe the circumstances that caused the injury, not the nature of the injury, and, therefore, are not used as a principal diagnosis. A maximum of five digits are used in coding the E Code. For example:

E948   Bacterial vaccines
E948.4   Tetanus
E948.5   Diphtheria

(DRG) Diagnosis-Related Grouping

Diagnosis-related groups (DRGs) are the basis for payment to hospitals under the Medicare Prospective Payment System (PPS). Originally developed at Yale University, DRGs, as adapted for use by Medicare, are intended to represent groups of hospital inpatients that are clinically similar to one another and relatively homogeneous with respect to financial resource use. (See Figure 4.21)

Payment Rates

The Health Care Financing Administration (HCFA) has established specific payment rates for each of approximately 477 DRGs. The special formula for calculating payment for a specific DRG is based on an individual hospital's blended PPS payment rate multiplied by the "cost weight" or "relative weight" of the DRG assigned to that care at the time of discharge. Generally, updates as to the list of DRGs and cost weights are issued by HCFA in September of each year.

DRG Assignment

Each Medicare patient discharge is assigned to only one DRG regardless of the number of services rendered or the number of days of care provided.

Figure 4.21   Diseases and Disorders of the
                    Circulatory System: Surgical Partitioning

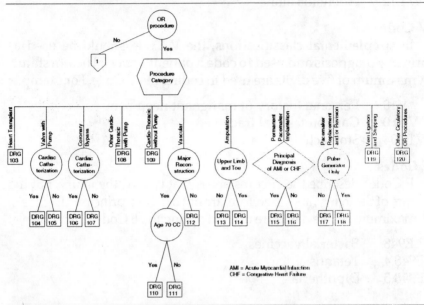

Lynch, Robert. "Reimbursement Management Primer for DRG and ICD-9 Analysis." *Journal of Cardiovascular Management*. 2(1):41-48, 1991.

First, the physician documents the patient's principal diagnosis, any additional diagnoses, and procedures performed. The hospital then records this information (in a timely manner) on the patient's bill using classifications and terminology consistent with the ICD-9-CM. The principal diagnosis, the principal procedure, and additional procedures as well as the patient's age, sex, and discharge status are reported to the hospital's request for payment. How the principal diagnosis can impact payment is demonstrated on figure 4.22.

The fiscal intermediary enters this information into its claims system and subjects the data to a series of automated screens called the Medicare Code Editor. Cases are then classified by a computer program ("Grouper") into the appropriate DRG.

Hospitals that are dissatisfied with the fiscal intermediary's decision regarding DRG assignment must request a review within 60 days after the date a claim is paid. The fiscal intermediary or the Peer Review Organization (PRO) then reviews the case and, if appropriate, changes the DRG classification.

Figure 4.22   Principal Diagnosis Impact on DRG Payment

DRG Classification
Principal DX-Impact on Payment

	Discharge summary attested DX	Review of chart supports
Principal DX	Angina pectoris	Intermediate coronary syndrome (unstable angina)
Secondary DX	ASHD Atrial fibrillation Hypothyroid Hypertension	ASHD Atrial fibrillation Hypothyroid Hypertension
Principle	Right/left heart cath	Right/left heart cath
DRG	125	124
Payment	$2158.99	$3,730.82

125—Circulatory disorders except AMI with cardiac cath without complex dx.

124—Circulatory disorders except AMI with cardiac cath and complex dx.

Note: More specific or complete information either in the principal diagnosis or secondary diagnosis position will change payment.

DRG Classification
Principal DX-Impact on Payment

	Discharge summary attested DX	Review of chart supports
Principal DX	Unstable angina	Unstable angina
Secondary DX	Myocardial infarction within 8 wk	Myocardial infarction (recent, acute)
Principal procedure	None	None
DRG	122	121
Payment	$3528.07	$5096.90

122 - Circulatory disorders with AMI and without CV complications, complex dx.

121 - Circulatory disorders with AMI and CV complications

Note: Recent myocardial infarction must have occurred within eight weeks of current admission to be applicable. Presence or absence of "cath" will not affect DRG.

Lynch, Robert. "Reimbursement Management Primer for DRG and ICD-9 Analysis." *Journal of Cardiovascular Management*. 2(1):41-48, 1990.

Procedure Coding—CPT-4 Current Procedural Terminology, Fourth Edition

The medical imaging department plays a major role in the CPT-4 coding process. Departments vary in their structure. However, in many departments, the clerk who first deals with the patient is responsible for assigning the correct code. The department charge master clearly displays the current CPT-4 in imaging services. It must be updated annually to reflect new procedures and delete obsolete procedures.

The American Medical Association publishes annually a CPT-4 full text available in paperback, magnetic computer tape, and disk. The purpose of the CPT-4 text is to provide a uniform language that will accurately describe medical, surgical, and diagnostic services and will thereby provide an effective means for reliable nationwide communication among physicians, patients, and third parties. This text may be purchased from: American Medical Association, 515 North State Street, Chicago, IL 60610.

It is important to point out that as of this writing, radiology codes include: Diagnostic Radiology, Nuclear Medicine, Radiation Oncology and Diagnostic Ultrasound—70010 to 79999. Most recently, the 1993 CPT-4 code book includes MRI codes as follows: 70336, 70540, 70551, 70552, 70553, 71550, 72141-72149, 72156-8, 72196, 73220, 73221, 73720, 73721, 74181 and 76400.

Because MRI has been considered experimental, some MRI claims have been denied reimbursement. Since March of 1991, Medicare has covered MRI procedures that include image components, such as surface coils, gating devices or paramagnetic contrast agents, provided that the service is reasonable and necessary.

Code Assignment

For your convenience the AMA has a "mini" edition of CPT codes; however, it is clearly pointed out that the user will need to refer to the unabridged edition of CPT text to locate those procedures not described in the abbreviated "mini" edition.

Each procedure or service is identified with a five digit code. For example:

Chest: 71020 Radiologic examination, chest, two views, frontal and lateral
71021 with apical lordotic procedure

71022   with oblique projections

71023   with fluoroscopy

It is paramount to remember to use additional codes that most accurately describe the service performed. For example, Special Services and Reports - 99070 for medical supplies used. You would add a supply code and describe items that are not customarily used to perform a study.

Finally, when listing procedures and services with unusual circumstances, the addition of the appropriate modifier code must be used. The modifier is recorded by a two-digit number placed after the usual CPT procedure number from which it is separated by a hyphen. Most often medical imaging departments will use either modifier -26 or 09926 to report the professional component. See figures 4.23 and 4.24 as illustrations of coding procedures.

Figure 4.23   An illustration of How to Use CPT Coding

For example:

A physician providing diagnostic or therapeutic radiology services, ultrasound or nuclear medicine services in a hospital would use either modifier -26 or 09926 to report the professional component.

For example:

74430-26 = Professional component only for cystography

or

74430 and 09926 = Professional component only for cystography

It's important to know the complete description of CPT code 74430 to fully understand how important this example is. The full description reads: *Cystography, minimum of three views; supervision and interpretation only.*

Did the CPT Advisory Committee choose a poor example here? It states "supervision and interpretation only," which implies a professional component. Isn't it redundant to use modifier -26 on this CPT code? Well, the committee didn't err. The example illustrates that in order to perform the procedure someone must provide technical support.

By not using modifier -26, a physician signals a third-party payer that a global service was provided and reimbursement is warranted for both components of the procedure. In short, the third party-payer is told that no one else will bill an aspect of this service.

For example, Dr. Weber, a radiologist, is partner in a group that owns a diagnostic imaging center. As is customary at the center, a urologist performs the injection portion of a cystogram while Dr. Weber provides supervision and interpretation. Dr. Weber would bill: 74430 *Cystography, minimum of three views; supervision and interpretation only.* Since modifier -26 is not used, the payer is notified that reimbursement for both components is warranted. Because of the separate nature of his services, the center's urologist is also entitled to reimbursement under 51600 *Injection procedure for cystography or voiding urethrocystography.*

Adapted from *Update*. Medi-Index Publications. Salt Lake City, Utah. 6(3):3,1991.

Figure 4.24   How Should Stereotactic Breast Biopsy be Coded?

Stereotactic breast biopsy (SBB) follows the general coding conventions associated with interventional radiology; namely, the procedure is comprised of a radiologic and surgical component. The radiology component is best reported as *either* code 76096 [Localization of breast nodule or calcification before operation, with market and confirmation of its position with appropriate imaging (radiologic or ultrasound)] or code 76090 (Mammography; unilateral). The unusual procedural service modifier (- 22) may be used in addition to codes 76096 or 76090 to account for the additional time and cost associated with stereotactic localization over and above that of conventional radiologic localization. Since a needle is used to collect the tissue sample, the breast needle biopsy code (19100) should be reported in addition to the radiologic code. An evaluation and management code may be billed if the patient visit/consultation conforms with stated CPT guidelines pertaining to such codes. Finally, code 99070 may be used to recoup costs incidental to the procedure (e.g. local anesthesia, compression pads, etc.)

Discussion:

Needle biopsy is a widely performed procedure for obtaining tissue samples from various parts of the body (e.g. breast, liver, prostate, etc.). Stereotactic localization, however, is relatively recent advance in breast biopsying. In stereotactic breast biopsy, mammograms are taken at different angles. When viewed stereotactically, the mammograms allow the suspicious area to be presented three dimensionally. Afterwards, with computer assistance, a core biopsy needle is able to be introduced into the abnormality from a biopsy device.

As compared to conventional breast biopsy, speed of the procedure is one benefit of SBB. A further benefit is the relatively pain-free nature of SBB. The three-dimensional representation of the tumor area enhances accuracy by minimizing the possibility that the needle misses the abnormality. Furthermore, breast biopsies in this fashion can be quickly scheduled and performed; therefore, delays in treatment can be minimized.

Turning to CPT coding of stereotactic breast biopsy, a specific code for the imaging associated with the procedure does not exist. However, CPT does include a code for breast needle biopsy (19100). As for the radiology component of the procedure, codes 76096 and 76090 are most analogous in terms of the type and extent of the imaging performed. Mammograms, as one form of localization technique, are inherent in code 76096; therefore, 76096 and 76090 are mutually exclusive. Stereotactic biopsy is relatively more physician and equipment intensive as compared to conventional mammographic localization. For these reasons, therefore, the (-22) modifier may be warranted. Contingent on CPT guidelines for evaluation and management codes, reporting the patient visit/consultation may be appropriate.

It has been suggested that in lieu of specific codes for stereotactic breast biopsy, either code 76360 (CT guidance for needle biopsy) or code 76355 (CT guidance for stereotactic localization) could be used for the radiologic component and the incisional breast biopsy code (19101) for the surgical component. In this instance, neither the CT codes nor the incisional biopsy code accurately represents the procedure being performed; as a consequence, they should not be used when billing for SBB. First of all, the imaging modality is plain film mammography, not CT. And second, incisional biopsy entails the laying open of the breast in order to directly remove tissue; clearly, it does not refer to core biopsy done through a simple skin nick (i.e. incision) done with a scalpel blade.

Adapted from: The RBMA Bulletin. November 1992, Costa Mesa, CA.

Healthcare Financing Administration's Common Procedural Coding System (HCPCS)

HCPCS ("hick-picks") is based on the American Medical Association's CPT-4 coding when reporting services under Medicare benefits. The HCPCS system has three levels of codes:

Level I   (CPT/HCPCS) AMA's CPT-4 codes.
Level II Physician and non-physician services not in CPT-4.
Level III Locally assigned codes are restricted to the series beginning with W, X, Y and Z.

Your intermediary will furnish you with Level II of the codes as appropriate, or you may purchase them at: U.S. Government Printing Office, Superintendent of Documents, Washington, D.C. 20402, Telephone 202/783-3232.

Billing Information

Briefly, in coding revenue codes, one must refer to up to three numeric digits to identify specific patient charges by types of services and by departments. For example, Therapeutic Nuclear Medicine (Service/Department)—342 (revenue code).

Further, the HCFA A-1450 (also known as the UB-82) is a uniform institutional provider bill suitable for use in billing multiple third-party payors. Electronic bill specifications may be implemented in lieu of HCFA-1450.

When billing multiple third parties, it is important to complete all items required by each payor who is to receive a copy. Instructions for completion are the same for inpatient and outpatient claims unless otherwise noted. See figure 4.25 Common Coding Errors.*

A Brief Explanation of "Cost Finding"

To determine how much reimbursement is due to a hospital from third-party payors, a cost determination occurs using a reimbursement formula. This cost determination or cost finding involves the allocation of overhead and indirect expenses to departments that produce revenue. Radiology is a great example of a revenue produc-

---

*Communicating Through Codes by Mary L. Wright, FAHRA, originally appeared in AHRA Radiology Reimbursement Reference: To Guide You Through the Maze of Radiology Reimbursement. AHRA. Sudbury, MA, 1991.

Figure 4.25   7 Most Common Reasons for Incorrect Radiology Reimbursement

1. Invalid CPT/HCPCS codes
2. CPT/HCPCS codes that don't describe the procedure performed
3. Billing descriptions that don't match the CPT code description
4. Use of a small number of codes to represent a large number of procedures
5. Charge ticket descriptions and codes that don't correlate with the chargemaster
6. Incorrect use of extra views, extra slices and room time
7. Incorrect use of unlisted or "99" codes

"7 Most Common Reasons for Incorrect Radiology Reimbursement" from *St. Anthony's Reimbursement Guide for Radiology Services.* Washington, D.C., 1992.

ing department, where laundry, maintenance, or medical records are examples of nonrevenue producing departments. The nonrevenue producing centers support the revenue producing departments and other support units in the hospital with essential hospital services. Through the cost-finding process a full costing-out of the price of doing business is figured by combining all of the direct costs associated with providing services with a prorated share of support or indirect costs. The allocation of costs in the cost-finding process can be done in several ways. The "step-down method" is the most straightforward method of cost allocation. In this method costs of nonrevenue producing centers are allocated to all other centers, both revenue and nonrevenue producing. Other cost finding processes include the double apportionment method, accumulative double apportionment, nonaccumulative double apportionment and integrated cost accounting. As more third-party payors establish payment methodologies that utilize new definitions of products and services, incentives to have information that efficiently relates costs to pricing become obvious.

For the most part, healthcare facilities run like most other business enterprises. Like other businesses, hospitals have fixed and variable costs. The percentage of fixed costs in hospitals is particularly high and that is normally due to the capital requirements and the labor intensive nature of healthcare as an industry. This high percentage of fixed costs is a significant factor for hospital managers to deal with and the effects of high fixed costs are especially a problem when there are decreases in the demand for services. Where a local factory can shut down for a few days or use temporary layoffs to offset reductions in business, a decrease in patient days in the average hospital cannot be reacted to quickly enough to have any significant effect on fixed expenses. If you work in a hospital, you will hear your administration talk about costs per patient day or FTEs per occupied bed. Top hospital management pays close attention to these ratios to prevent an upward creep in fixed expenses.

You will hear numerous other financial terms used on a regular basis during discussions of the hospital's financial situation. What follows here is a brief discussion of other hospital economic factors:

- Depreciation: Millions of dollars are invested in capital assets in hospitals. Through a depreciation schedule these capital investments are allocated and then recovered over their useful life. An allowance for depreciation of assets used in providing services to patients is an allowable cost for reimbursement purposes when the depreciation is properly accounted for.
- Interest: Interest occurred in indebtedness is an allowable cost for reinbursement purposes if the interest on a loan made to satisfy a financial need is strictly related to patient care.
- Bad debt, charity, and courtesy discounts: These are not usually allowed as costs. These items may be treated as deductions from gross revenues.
- Cash flow: As mentioned in the introduction of this discussion of healthcare finance, accounts receivable is the largest component of a hospital's working capital. Along with fixed assets, it is also the other largest single asset a hospital may have. Seventy to eighty percent of current assets may be held in accounts receivable. The management of accounts receivable is a complicated endeavor that will begin prior to admission with preadmission screening and financial counseling. Minimizing the amount of cash in accounts receivable is accomplished through control of the length of the accounts receivable payment cycle. The shorter the cycle, the less cash is held up in accounts receivable. When days in accounts receivable begin to lengthen and total accounts receivable dollars become excessive, cash flow problems occur. The number of days in accounts receivable by payor class is closely watched by senior management. As a benchmark, fifty-five days is considered to be highly desirable as an overall average for collection.

Understanding the Medicare Cost Report

The process for determining the cost of providing services to Medicare recipients is the documentation required of all healthcare institutions that participate in the Medicare program. This understanding of the real costs of providing a service is a very enlightening exercise. First, let's take a very unsophisticated look at department revenues versus expenses. Suppose for a moment that your department posted $3 million in gross charges last year. You know that your personnel expenses and nonpersonnel expenses total less than $750,000. Factor in that you have a pro-rata share of utilities and other support services. Is it fair to conclude that the approximately $2 million in excess revenues over expenses are profit? Don't be lulled into believing that your radiology department is some enormous cash generating machine! Sit down with a financial manager in your organization and learn the cold, cruel facts of healthcare accounting. You may be shocked to learn that the hospital only collects 42 percent of your department's gross billings.

The Medicare cost report is a very complicated piece of data. To help you develop an understanding of this cost report, what follows is a very simple explanation of the mechanics of this important process.

Medicare does not simply accept the fact that a cost has occurred as a justification for reimbursement. Tests of reasonableness, necessity, and prudence are used by Medicare in order to determine the level of reimbursement that you will receive for the services provided to patients in your facility. Medicare has used a cost reimbursement system for over 25 years. *The Health Insurance Manual 15* (HIM15) is the provider reimbursement manual that describes the process for cost finding. A simplified overview of the process of completing the Medicare cost report is described here.

The Medicare Cost Report is completed by using a series of worksheets, A through H, that is filed within 90 days of the conclusion of the cost-reporting period (usually your fiscal year end). The process of completing the cost report is serial because information entered on each worksheet is dependent on calculations on preceding or supplemental worksheets. If you have completed a long-form income tax report for the IRS, you can only begin to grasp an understanding for the detail required for Medicare cost accounting.

Worksheet A categorizes the array of services provided by your institution and their direct costs. Worksheet B is used to calculate indirect costs. The process used in order to calculate these costs are statistical bases such as square feet of space used, cost of equipment, pounds of laundry, meals served, and so forth. Worksheet B allocates the costs of nonrevenue producing cost centers to revenue producing cost centers. When all the nonrevenue cost centers have been allocated to revenue producing cost centers, these costs are then carried over to Worksheets C and D. The purpose of Worksheet C is to develop a cost-to-charge ratio. The method of determining the cost-to-charge ratio is to take total costs in all ancillary services and divide them by total charges. On Worksheet D, Medicare's charges are then multiplied by this cost-to-charge ratio developed in Worksheet C to determine what Medicare costs are in the program. Worksheet E develops total costs of Medicare services, comparing them to total Medicare charges. Schedules A-E complete the hospital portion of the cost reporting. Medicare, by regulation, will pay the lower of either the cost or the charge. Because Medicare will pay the lower of either the cost or the charge, the provider needs to insure that charges to Medicare exceed their costs. Understanding the mechanics of cost reporting is important to the radiology manager if he expects to be able to effectively interact with senior management relative to reimbursement issues in imaging services.

Budgeting Basics

The long-term strategic financial plan dictates a direction for the future that is driven by a yearly budgeting exercise. Budgeting along with strategic planning establishes the organization's goals and policies that are translated into the management objectives for each department. Financial objectives for the department are reflected in dollars and in nonmonetary statistical units. Through the budgeting process, hospital managers take a close look at departmental operations and the major activities of the organization as a whole. When you submit your budget to upper administration, it will be consolidated into a final budgeting plan for the entire organization.

There are two general approaches to preparing budgets. **Zero-based** and **historical-continuous expense budgeting** are the two methods that you will see most often in healthcare organizations. With the zero-based budgeting approach, the actual expense information necessary to formulate the budget is calculated by starting with nothing and adding the expenses necessary to build the budget for an entire year. Zero-based budgeting is a great learning experience for the novice budgeter because it is like building a house one stud at a time. Like the ingredients needed in order to bake a cake, the zero-based budgeting process looks at the end product from the standpoint of the sum of its parts. The historical-continuous budgeting method is much easier to do. With historical-continuous budgeting, it is assumed that you will spend at least what you did last year. This assumption is totally based on the premise that the previous data is accurate and forecasts for future volumes will meet budget calculations. In actuality, most radiology managers use a combination of the zero-based and historical-continuous expense budgeting processes.

In most organizations the budget process is an annual rite of spring that grabs middle management in much the same feverish pitch that preparation for Joint Commission entails. As a department manager you will enter a period of solitary confinement where you will create your annual department budgets. You will then defend these budgets in front of an organizational budget committee. This budget committee operates as a tribunal and your interview with the budget committee will likely involve a long and detailed review of each line item of your budget. Zero-based budgeting requires that the entire budget be defended each year because the zero-based budget is based on the premise that all activities are new. Historical-continuous expense budgets are incremental in nature and the defense of such budgets is much easier. When explaining why certain line items exceed historical expenditures, the increases over the last year's budget are defended based on what is expected to occur in the new year.

The Operating Budget

Management will develop and review a formal system of budget preparation that is uniform for the entire organization. The first step in the budget process for your organization, if it is a hospital, is to make the following projections for each department:

1. Forecast anticipated admissions and patient days.
2. Forecast anticipated admissions and patient days per nursing unit.
3. Forecast work units for all volume dependent departments.

The operating budget is summarized in the hospital's income statement and is usually prepared using an accrual method of accounting. Expense of revenue over expenses is the hospital's "bottom line," and a positive bottom line is the goal of the budget.

Cash Budget

A cash budget is prepared by converting operations budgets from an accrual basis to a cash basis. Projecting cash flow is vital to the survival of the organization because cash flow means being able to meet payroll, pay creditors, and avoid borrowing short-term capital. Receivables from inpatient and outpatient services are major sources of cash. In addition to patient revenues, the hospital will estimate other operating revenue such as cafeteria food sales, parking charges, gift shop revenues, and nonoperating revenues such as donations, interest income, and sales and proceeds from the sales of assets.

Capital Budget

The hospital must continue to provide services to patients in a manner that is technologically efficient and competitive with other providers. If the organization expects to survive into the future, it must adequately invest in facilities and equipment. Such factors as community needs, marketability, urgency, and competitive pressures all impact the decision-making process for acquiring new capital equipment.

The Final Budget

Once you have turned your budget in and it has been merged with all other departmental budgets, the senior management team will review and revise the total organization's budget to meet the bottom line dictated by the strategic financial plan. Management will compare the final cash budget with the operating and capital budgets to gauge anticipated profitability. When available cash falls short of expected expenditures, then management must face the difficult task of finding ways to cut expenses and increase revenues. When cash falls short of expected expenditures, usually a second round of budget committee reviews will occur. It is during the second round of budget reviews that your budget committee will begin to look very closely at education and travel, and supply management. FTEs will also be closely scrutinized and discussions of productivity will lead to suggested new efficiencies.

According to Stephen F. Nowak, one of the traditional problems faced by radiology managers is reconciliation of department expenditures with the department budget. Nowak makes some suggestions on preparing the radiology budget. These suggestions are summarized here:

1. Zero-based budgeting is less biased but is more time consuming to prepare than the historical-continuous budget.
2. Accurately anticipate future workload activity by collecting five years of information and study the levels of change from year to year.
3. Know the procedure mix for your department as well as the patient referral sources for each procedure.
4. Categorize expenditures in the proper accounts. Avoid spending dollars from one account for materials that should have been purchased from another account. This practice will only unfavorably weight your expense accounts and throw off your historical utilization statistics.
5. Negotiate the best terms possible for large volume purchases, capital equipment acquisitions, and maintenance agreements.
6. Limit the quantities of materials on hand in the department. Avoid situations of over stocking, particularly new items that haven't established a track record for use yet.

Conclusion

This discussion of basic financial management was designed to introduce and review basic managerial finance principles as they relate to the operation of the radiology department. An important management tool is the departmental budget. Besides creating cost awareness and operationalizing department goals, a budget is used to evaluate performance and to identify inefficiencies in the way the department functions. In today's competitive healthcare environment, financial planning and budgeting are essential managerial skills for radiology managers. The appendices of this chapter contain financial and reimbursement terms of interest to the radiology manager. The following textbooks are suggested resources for radiology managers who would like to study the subject of healthcare finance in greater detail.

Suggested Resources

Donald F. Beck. *Basic Hospital Financial Management*, 2nd ed. Rockville, Maryland: Aspen Publishers, Inc., 1989.

William O. Cleverly. *Essentials of Health Care Finance*, 2nd ed. Rockville, Maryland: Aspen Publishers, Inc., 1986.

Allen G. Herkimer, Jr. *Understanding Health Care Budgeting*. Rockville, Maryland: Aspen Publishers, Inc., 1988.

Bruce R. Neumann, James D. Suver, and William N. Zelman. *Financial Management: Concepts and Applications for Health Care Providers*, 2nd ed. Owings Mill, Maryland: National Health Publishing, 1988.

Appendix A   Glossary of Financial Terms*

Budget   Document that identifies the expected resources and expenditures for a given future period and reflects the nature and source of these resources and expenditures.

Controllable cost   A cost that is directly influenced by a given manager within a given time span.

Cost accounting   Accumulation and communication, in conformity with generally accepted principles, of historical and projected economic data relating to the financial position and operating results of an enterprise. Used as a tool for decision making.

---

*Adapted from Steve F. Kukla. *Cost Accounting and Financial Analysis for the Hospital Administrator*. American Hospital Publishing, Inc. 1986.

Cost allocation (or cost apportionment)   The assignment to each of several institutional departments or services of an equitable proportion of the costs of activities that serve all of them.

Cost center   Organizational unit for which revenue and expenses are accumulated separately in the accounts.

Cost-to-charge ratio   The proportional relationship of Medicare cost to total cost applied to total charges in a hospital operating department for Medicare cost-finding purposes.

Diagnosis-related group (DRG)   Patient classification system relating demographic, diagnostic, and therapeutic characteristics of patients to length of inpatient stay and amount of resources consumed.   Provides a framework for specifying hospital case mix. A system that identifies classifications of illnesses and injuries for which Medicare payment is made as part of the prospective payment program.

DRG weight   An index number that reflects the relative resource consumption associated with each DRG.

Differential cost (or incremental cost)   The difference between the total cash outlay necessary to operate the company if a proposed action is taken and the total outlay required by the alternative the company will accept if the proposal is rejected.

Direct labor   All labor that is physically traceable to the finished goods in an economically feasible manner.

Direct material   All material that is physically observable as being identified with the finished goods and that can be traced to the finished goods in an economically feasible manner.

Discharge   A patient who is formally released from the hospital, dies in the hospital, or is transferred to another hospital or unit that is excluded from the prospective pricing system.

Fee for service   Method of charging patients for services or treatment in which a provider bills for each patient encounter or treatment or service rendered.

Fixed cost   A cost that remains unchanged in total for a given time period, despite wide fluctuations in activity, and becomes progressively smaller on a per-unit basis as production increases.

Full cost The direct, indirect, controllable, and noncontrollable costs associated with each organizational unit or cost center.

General ledger The main file of accounts containing data on the assets, liabilities and owner's equity of the company.

Gross margin The margin between sales revenue and the cost of the merchandise that was sold.

GROUPER Computer software program that is used by the fiscal intermediary to assign discharges to the appropriate DRGs using the following information abstracted from the inpatient bill: patient's age and sex, principal diagnosis, principal procedures performed, and discharge status.

Major diagnosis Diagnosis accounting for the greatest resource consumption during a patient stay.

Major diagnostic category (MDC) Grouping of patients into major clinical categories based on organ systems and disease etiology. The 23 MDCs include the listing of diagnoses that appear in the International Classification of Diseases, 9th Revision, Clinical Modification (ICD-9-CM).

Management by exception To focus attention on areas where anticipated costs vary.

Marginal cost The change in total cost associated with a change in the quantity of output per period of time.

Medical record Record of a patient, maintained by a hospital or a physician for the purpose of documenting clinical data on diagnosis, treatment, and outcome.

Medical specialty The grouping of specific areas of medicine, (e.g., dermatology, ophthalmology, neurology).

Medicare Federal program, created by Title XVIII- Health Insurance for the Aged - a 1965 amendment to the Social Security Act that provides health insurance benefits primarily to persons over the age of 65 and others eligible for Social Security benefits.

Operating margin That portion of net income attributable to the excess of operating revenue over operating expense.

Overhead Indirect costs that are not traceable to individual jobs.

Part A, Medicare   Hospital Insurance Program, the compulsory portion of Medicare, that automatically enrolls all persons aged 65 and over entitled to benefits under Old Age, Survivors, Disability and Health Insurance Program or railroad retirement, persons under 65 who have been eligible for disability for more than two years, and insured workers (and their dependents) requiring hemodialysis or kidney transplantation.

Part B, Medicare   Supplementary Medical Insurance Program, the voluntary portion of Medicare, that includes physician's services and in which all persons entitled to Part A, the Hospital Insurance Program, may enroll on a monthly premium basis.

Patient billing   Charging of patients for care rendered.

Preferred provider organization   Payment arrangement organized by hospitals, physicians, insurers, employers or third-party administrators in which designated healthcare providers negotiate with group purchasers to provide healthcare services for a defined population at a discount rate in return for prompt payment and an expectation of an increased volume of patients; in which providers are usually paid on a fee-for-service basis and are not at risk for the use of services by the defined population; and in which subscribers can select any provider for care, but are given economic or other incentives to use the designated hospitals or physicians.

Price variance (or rate variance)   Difference between actual and standard input prices for a specified quantity of resource inputs.

Prime cost   Direct materials and direct labor.

Product cost   Total amount of cost assigned to a particular product or job order.

Product costing   Process of measuring the costs of end-product activities.

Product line   Specific individual goods manufactured and sold in an organizational unit.

Prospective payment   Method of third-party payment by which rates of payment to providers for services to patients are established in advance for the coming fiscal year, and providers are paid these rates for services delivered regardless of the costs actually incurred in providing these services.

Quantity variance   Difference between actual and standard input quantities for the output actually achieved.

Rate per diem   Established rate of payment determined by dividing the total cost of providing routine inpatient services for a given period by the total number of inpatient days of care provided during that period.

Reimbursement, cost-based   by a third-party payor to a hospital of all allowable costs incurred by the hospital in the provision of services to patients covered by the contract.

Relative value unit (RVU)   A weighted work load measurement based on the relative time, resources, and skill required to produce a product.

Responsibility accounting   An accounting system that accumulates and communicates revenue, expense, and statistical data based on established organizational units responsible for producing the revenue and incurring the expenses.

Standard cost   Management's estimate, prepared in advance, of the cost of the inputs that should be necessary to obtain a specific material, product or service.   Target cost.

Utilization statistic   Measurement of the use of a product.

Variable cost   A given cost that changes in total in proportion to changes in activity.

Variance   Difference between actual results and the results embodied in performance standards.

Appendix B—Glossary of Reimbursement Terms*

Admitting diagnosis   The diagnosis recorded at the time of admission as a basis for examination and treatment of the patient.

Ancillary services   Diagnostic and/or therapeutic services provided by the hospital (e.g., respiratory therapy, radiology).

---

*Adapted from "Communicating Through Codes" by Mary L. Wright, FAHRA originally appeared in *AHRA Radiology Reimbursement Reference: To Guide You Through the Maze of Radiology Reimbursement*. AHRA. Sudbury, MA, 1991.

Appeals   Most disputes between hospitals and the federal government about the prospective payment system must be resolved by administrative or judicial appeals. The Provider Reimbursement Review Board hears administrative appeals. The scope of review is limited. Any successful appeal would be applied to the next cost reporting period after the decision is issued. However, hospitals that successfully appeal their base year cost calculations will receive a retroactive adjustment. The appeal is allowed only if the fiscal intermediary was "unreasonable and clearly erroneous" in determining the base year costs using the data then available.

Assignment   The patient can legally sign away his right to receive reimbursement from the insurance payor, thus, giving that right to the physician or hospital. The insurer issues the check directly to the healthcare provider. The amount paid depends on the patient's policy provisions.

Assignment under Medicare rules   Patient may "assign" their right to receive insurance paid amounts to the physician. Physicians agreeing to "accept assignment" (participating physicians) agree to accept Medicare's calculated reimbursement rate as payment in full and guarantee not to balance bill. The physician is reimbursed directly by Medicare, and can charge patients only for the $75 deductible and 20 percent co-insurance based on Medicare's payment level. Physicians who do not accept assignment bill patients directly and can charge more than the Medicare reimbursement level. A 1987 law placed restrictions on the charging practices of nonparticipating radiologists. Their charges are limited to 115 percent of the RVS charge for the procedure.

Average length of stay (ALOS)   The average length of hospitalization of inpatients discharged during the period under consideration.

Balance Billings   The practice of holding a patient liable for payment of any fee in excess of the amount paid by the insurers. Medicare patients can only be held liable for amounts up to the level set by the 1987 law. When a service is not a covered benefit by Medicare, the patient can be billed for the full amount if the patient signs a statement for that amount **prior** to receiving care.

Base year costs   During the three-year phase-in of prospective payment, part of a hospital's payments is based on hospital-specific costs. To arrive at the hospital's average costs for Medicare discharge, base year cost data are used. The base year is a hospital's cost reporting period ending on or after September 30, 1982, and before September 30, 1983. The costs are updated through fiscal 1984 to account for inflation. The costs that are "passed through" prospective payment can't be included in a hospital's base year costs.

Blue Cross and Blue Shield A network of nonprofit and mutual health insurance organizations that offer insurance plans providing benefits for a range of healthcare services. Hospitals and physicians may choose to sign BCBS contracts as Preferred Providers. These negotiated contracts set maximum fees that will be paid for services to patients covered by the BCBS plan. Many Blue Cross organizations offer HMO plan alternative also.

Capital-related costs These costs include depreciation expenses, taxes, leases and rentals, the costs of betterments and improvements, costs of minor equipment, insurance expenses on depreciation assets, interest expenses, the capital-related costs of related organizations, and a return on equity for investor-owned providers.

Carriers Carriers are agencies contracting with Health Care Financing Administration (HCFA) to administer Part B services. These groups have more discretion in policy than Fiscal Intermediaries.

Case A term synonymous with discharge.

Case mix A diagnosis-specific measure of the length of stay, cost, complexity, and intensity of services provided by a hospital.

Case mix index To eliminate any variations in a hospital's base year costs that are attributable to the complexity of cases it treated, the hospital's base year costs are divided by the 1981 fiscal year case mix index. The index is a statistic that represents the costliness of each hospital's mix of cases compared with the national average case mix.

CHAMPUS Government sponsored programs to provide hospital and medical services for dependents to active, deceased, and retired armed forces personnel when military services are not available.

Charges Prices assigned to units of medical services, such as a visit to a physician or a day in the hospital. Charges for services may not be related to the actual costs of providing the services.

Charges, actual The amount a physician or other practitioner actually bills a patient for a particular medical service or provider for a given service.

Charges, allowable Generic term referring to the maximum fee that a third party will use in reimbursing a provider for a given service.

Co-insurance As a feature of most health insurance plans for physician services, patients are asked to pay a portion (usually 20 percent) of billed charges. These are assessed after the deductible is paid.

Commerical insurance Commerical insurers represent more than 1,000 large and small for-profit insurers and Administered Services Only (ASO) businesses that write health insurance coverage, primarily for employee groups. Leading firms are Aetna, Travelers, Prudential, and so forth. Traditionally, commercial insurers are indemnity payers, and contribute either a fixed amount or a percentage of charges for physicians' services.

Comorbidity A pre-existing condition which, in addition to a patient's principal diagnosis, would presumably extend the length of hospitalization by at least one day in approximately 75 percent of the cases.

Complication A condition which develops subsequent to a patient's admission and would predictably extend the length of hospitalization by at least one day in approximately 75% of the cases.

Costs Expenses incurred in the provision of goods or services.

Costs, allowable Items or elements of an institution's costs that are reimbursable under a payment formula.

Coverage Refers to the status of medical services as specific benefits offered under an insurance plan. For example, some plans "cover" maternity care but do not "cover" high risk nursery services. Others cover ophthalmology exams but not optometry services. Note: Coverage does NOT ensure payment; there may be requirements for pre-certification or medical necessity clauses. Also, coverage does not say anything on the issues of reimbursement amounts.

CPT-4 Common Procedural Terminology, Fourth Edition. Five digit codes used to report procedures. Each code stands for a very specific description of services performed. The codes are defined by the AMA and the volume is revised annually.

Deductible A feature of most health insurance plans for physician services. Patients are asked to pay a certain dollar level of costs upfront before any insurance payments begin. For example, deductibles for Medicare part B are the first $100 per year, and in many Blue Shield plans it is the first $100 per family member.

Direct medical education costs These are the costs of approved medical education activities. Only costs for medical education programs operated directly by the hospital will be excluded from the prospective payment system.

Discharge This is the formal release of the patient from the hospital. A discharge results in payment of the full DRG rate.

Discharge status Disposition of the patient on discharge (i.e., home, expired, left AMA, transferred to SNF).

Diagnostic related groupings (DRGs) Numerical codes, each designating a broad grouping of diseases primarily by body systems. A single payment level is attached to each and relates to reimbursement for inpatient hospital stays. DRG levels can be increased by complicating (co-morbidity) diagnoses, particularly when more than one body system is effected.

DRG cost weights Each DRG is assigned a number, or weight, that reflects its resource utilization. The weight is multiplied by the average cost for a Medicare discharge to arrive at the payment for the particular DRG.

DRGs 468, 469, 470 These three DRGs don't group illnesses but are used for administrative purposes. DRG 468 includes all patients who had a surgical procedure performed that was unrelated to their MDC. For example, a patient may be admitted for cataract surgery but suffer a heart attack while in the hospital and have a coronary bypass operation instead. DRG 469 is a discharge that has been assigned a diagnosis that isn't the principal diagnosis. An example is a diagnosis of diabetes for a pregnant patient who actually was admitted for her pregnancy, not her diabetes. The fiscal intermediary will return a claim for DRG 469 and ask the provider to enter the correct principal diagnosis. DRG 470 is a discharge with invalid data. Again, the fiscal intermediary will return the claim to the hospital for more data.

DRG coordinator   A full-time hospital employee who is responsible for coordinating management activities relative to reimbursement systems.

DRG creep   Assignment and sequencing of diagnosis and procedures based on resource consumption to maximize reimbursement.

DRG Rate   A fixed-dollar amount based on an average of all patients in a specific DRG in the base year, adjusted for inflation, economic factors, and bad debt.

Explanation of medicare benefits (EOMB)   A form letter returned to a Medicare patient by the carrier following the submission of a Medicare claim. The EOMB outlines the carrier's decision regarding coverage and reimbursement of the services billed for and the reasons why coverage or reimbursement may have been denied.

Excluded providers   Some facilities are excluded from prospective payment. They include alcohol and drug treatment, psychiatric and rehabilitative hospitals and units, as well as children's and long-term care hospitals. Hospitals in Maryland, Massachusetts, New Jersey and New York—states having alternative payment programs for Medicare—also are excluded from prospective payment. Except for hospitals in these four states, excluded hospitals are paid on a reasonable costs basis subject to TEFRA Limits.

Federal rate   Until October 1, 1986, the hospital-specific rate is blended with a federal rate to arrive at a hospital's payment. In the first year, 25 percent of the payment is based on the federal rate; in the second year, 50 percent; and in the third year, 75 percent. By the fourth year, the hospital's payment is based solely on the federal rate, which is adjusted each October. The federal rate is a combination of the regional and national rates. This blend changes each year. In the first year, 100 percent of the federal rate is based on the regional rate; the second year, 75 percent of the regional rate and 25 percent is the national rate; the third year it's a 50-50 split; in the fourth year 100 percent is the national rate. That means that in the fourth year, all hospitals will be receiving the same basic payment rate.

Federal employee program (FEP)   Policies to cover federal government employees (who are not Medicare beneficiaries). Participating companies are free to develop their own fee schedule for reimbursement. Benefits are consistent; amount paid may vary.

Fiscal intermediary (FI)   The agency that is responsible for reimbursement intervention between hospitals and the Healthcare Financing Administration.

Final diagnosis   Can be any of the diagnoses recorded after all data is accumulated during the course of the patient's hospitalization. The final diagnosis differs from the principal diagnosis.

Global fee   Payment made for both the professional and technical components of procedures. Physicians performing diagnostic radiology procedures in their offices or at freestanding imaging centers will submit one bill and be paid one global fee.

GROUPER   The federal government's fiscal intermediary will assign a DRG to a discharge using the Grouper computer software program. This program screens information from the inpatient bill to assign the DRG. The DRG criteria include the patient's age, sex, principal diagnosis, secondary diagnoses, procedures performed, and discharge status. The program may be bought from Health Systems International, New Haven, CT.

Healthcare Financing Administration (HCFA)   The federal agency within the Department of Health and Human Services (DHHS) that administers the Medicare program.

HCPCS   A system of codes based on CPT-4, but supplemented with additional codes for nonphysician services. The system was developed by the Health Care Financing Administration for use in Medicare billing.

HMO   A Health Maintenance Organization is a special type of joint insurance/medical care program. Enrollees pay the HMO a fixed annual premium and receive all needed medical services at no (or nominal) additional out-of-pocket cost. Patients are usually limited to receiving care from a group of HMO hospitals and doctors. Almost 30 million Americans are in HMOs, which are managed much like private insurance companies but have internal policy making processes to establish medical protocols and services covered.

Hospital-specific rate   This is the portion of a hospital's payment that's based on a hospital's base year costs per discharge, divided by the case mix index, updated for inflation and adjusted for the specific DRG. In the first year of the system, 75 percent of the payment is based on the hospital-specific rate; in the second year, 50 percent; and in the third year, 25 percent. The hospital-specific rate is adjusted at the beginning of each hospital's fiscal year.

ICD9-CM   International Classification of Diseases, 9th Edition, Clinical Modifications. The World Health Organization developed this system of codes to describe illnesses, symptoms, accidental causes and diagnoses. The books are revised approximately every 10 years. These 3 to 5 digit codes are used to explain the condition causing a patient's need for healthcare services.

Indirect medical education costs   Hospitals are given additional payments for the indirect medical education costs attributable to an approved graduate medical education program. These costs include the additional tests and procedures that residents might order during the education process. Payment is based on the number of interns and residents employed at a hospital. If the interns and residents work at a hospital but aren't on the hospital's payroll, the hospital must have a long-standing relationship with the employing hospital to be paid for the costs generated by these medical students.

Industrial workers compensation plans   Insures against on-the-job injury or illness. Employer pays the premium. Each state's Industrial Commission has laws governing these plans, frequently including fee schedules.

Major diagnostic categories   DRGs fall into 23 MDCs. Each MDC corresponds to a single organ system or combination of any organ system and disease etiology. MDCs are further sub-divided based on whether the patient received a medical or surgical procedure.

Medicaid   A joint federal/state health insurance program for the poor and medically indigent. This program is administered differently in each state, and it has fairly tight restrictions of payments for physician services and drugs.

Medical review entities   Fiscal intermediaries, professional standards review organizations, and eventually, peer review organizations will undertake all inpatient hospital medical review. They are responsible for determining the medical necessity, appropriateness, and quality of care as well as validating the DRG classification. The medical review entity also will review a hospital's admission practices to determine whether admission rates have increased or the number of short stay cases has increased. Under prospective payment, hospitals may have an incentive to admit patients unnecessarily or to discharge a patient early. Hospitals are expected to contract with PROs to conduct the medical review. A hospital's DRG payment will be contingent on having a contract with a PRO.

Medically unnecessary services and custodial care When a physician discharges a patient but the patient chooses not to leave the hospital, the hospital may bill the beneficiary for these custodial days of care or for noncovered services. The beneficiary must be notified in writing that he or she will be billed. Also, the Medicare fiscal intermediary must concur with the hospital's determination that the services aren't covered by the Medicare program.

Medicare A federally sponsored health insurance program available to all social security beneficiaries. Medicare has two separate programs—Part A covers hospital inpatient care; Part B covers physician and outpatient care.

Medigap A private insurance policy purchased independently by Medicare beneficiaries to "fill the coverage/reimbursement gaps" in Medicare. Medigap policies frequently pay for coinsurance not picked up by Medicare, and in some circumstances cover services excluded by Medicare such as outpatient drugs.

Operating room (OR) procedure Procedures performed in a fully equipped operating room or those procedures determined as significant in terms of degree of risk or resource consumption, as contrasted with a "non-OR procedure".

"OR" procedure hierarchy Ranking of all "OR" resource consumption. "OR" procedures are ranked from left to right on the tree diagrams with priority given to left-most procedures. Also referred to as "surgical hierarchy."

Other diagnoses All conditions that coexist at the time of admission, develop subsequently, or affect the treatment received or the length of stay. Diagnoses that relate to an earlier episode and have no bearing on the current hospital stay should be excluded. Postoperative, medical, or other complications arising during the stay should be recorded.

Other procedures Those performed during the principal operative episode or during the length of stay, which may include diagnostic or exploratory procedures. These may include significant procedures that carry an operative or personnel or special facilities or equipment cost.

Outliers Hospitals get additional payments for cases involving unusually costly cases, called cost outliers. Payments have been set aside for outliers by taking 5.7 percent of the budget for regional and national rates.

Participating physicians A feature of the Medicare program and many Blue Shield plans where providers sign a contract to accept the insurer's price as payment in full for services rendered to subscribers.

Pass-through costs Allowable costs that are reimbursed in the hospital's Medicare cost report and are not subject to the limits. Examples are capital costs (depreciation, interest, rent) and approved education costs. Capital-related costs and direct medical education costs will be reimbursed on a cost basis until the federal government devises a formula to include reimbursement for these expenditures in prospective payment.

Ping-ponging Deliberate transfer of a patient between hospitals to maximize reimbursement.

Pre-admission testing Diagnostic services provided to outpatients prior to their scheduled hospitalization.

Preferred provider organizations (PPO) A group of providers who have an agreement with either an employer or insurance company to offer medical services on a fee-for-service basis at a discounted rate.

Principal diagnosis Condition established after study to be chiefly responsible for occasioning the admission of the patient to the hospital for care.

Principal procedure One performed for definitive treatment rather than one performed for diagnostic or exploratory purposes, or was necessary to take care of a complication. The principal procedure is that most related to principal diagnosis.

Professional component That portion of a payment reimbursing for a physician's services. For diagnostic radiology procedures this generally means supervision of the x-ray process and interpretation of the results.

Professional review organization (PRO) An organization which contracts with hospitals to perform a review of the quality, necessity, and appropriateness of care rendered to health insurance beneficiaries.

Prospective Payment Medicare will pay hospitals a fixed price per discharge for each diagnosis-related group of illnesses. These prices are paid regardless of a hospital's costs or charges. Rates for computing the DRG prices will be updated annually. They must be proposed by June 1 and finalized by Sept. 1. A hospital converts to prospective payment when it starts a new cost reporting period on or after October 1, 1983.

Prospective payment assessment commission This independent advisory group will suggest changes in DRG payment rates to the Department of Health and Human Services.

Referral centers Rural hospitals with 500 or more beds will have their rates adjusted by the urban regional and national rates rather than by the rural rates. Other hospitals must meet certain criteria to qualify as a referral hospital, although HHS' Healthcare Financing Administration hasn't yet decided what the adjustment to the rate will be. These hospitals must admit 50 percent of their Medicare patients as referrals from other hospitals or by referral from physicians not on the hospital's medical staff. Also, at least 60 percent of their Medicare patients must be furnished to beneficiaries who live more than 25 miles from the hospital.

Regional rate This is the average cost of treating a Medicare patient in each of the nine census divisions. In each region, an urban and rural rate are determined. Each of these rates has labor and nonlabor-related portions. The average regional rate is adjusted to reflect a hospital's wage index, outliers and the DRG weight.

Reimbursement Refers to the mechanisms for calculating payments, and the subsequent payments made by insurers for covered services.

Reimbursement, cost-based   The amount of the payment based on the costs to the provider of delivering the service.   The actual payment may be based on any one of several different formulas such as full cost, full cost plus an additional percentage, allowable costs, or a fraction of costs.

Reimbursement, prospective   A payment method in which hospital rates are set prospectively before services are rendered, and are based upon expected classes and volumes of patients.

Reimbursement, retrospective   Payment is provided by a third-party carrier for costs or charges actually incurred by subscribers in a previous time period.

Sole community hospitals   During the transition period, these hospitals may elect to be paid a prospective rate based 75 percent on the hospital-specific rate and 25 percent on the regional rate.   To qualify as a sole community hospital, a facility must meet any of four criteria: (1) have no other hospital within a 10 mile radius; (2) have no other hospital within a 25-to-50 mile radius and have no more than 15% of the residents in its service area using another hospital or no other hospital is accessible, because of weather conditions or geography, for more than one month a year; (3) have no other hospitals within 15-to-25 miles and weather conditions or geography make other hospitals inaccessible for more than one month a year; and (4) have less than 50 beds and have no other hospitals within a 25-to-50 mile radius. Urban hospitals may seek sole community hospital status in unusual situations when the hospital is the sole source of inpatient services and is in a remote section of a large county.

Technical component   That portion of a payment reimbursing for nonphysician (i.e., professional component) supplies and services. For diagnostic radiology procedures, this traditionally involves x-ray film, use of the x-ray machine and facilities, contrast media, services of a radiology technician, and so forth.

TEFRA   *Tax Equity and Fiscal Responsibility Act* of 1982.

Transfer   A patient is considered a transfer when he or she is moved from one unit of the hospital to another; is transferred to another hospital receiving prospective payments; is transferred to a hospital that is in Maryland, Massachusetts, New Jersey, or New York; or is transferred to a hospital that hasn't switched to prospective payment yet. The hospital transferring the patient is paid a per diem amount; the discharging hospital will be paid the full prospective payment rate for the patient. The federal government intends eventually to pay only the discharging hospital.

Third-party A general concept referencing a health insurance program (e.g., Medicare, Medicaid, Blue Cross, etc.) that pays doctors or hospitals for medical services provided to patients.

Unbundling This is the practice of billing under Part B of the Medicare program for nonphysician services provided to a hospital inpatient. As of October 1, 1983, hospitals are prohibited from unbundling. Only physician services provided to inpatients may be billed under Part B. Lab and radiology services furnished to a hospital's inpatients also are subject to the unbundling prohibition. One exception to the unbundling provision is that physicians can continue to bill Part B for services provided by certified registered nurse anesthetists. The exception only applies during the first three years of prospective payments. To qualify, the physician must have employed the nurse anesthetist for the hospital's cost reporting period ending before September 30, 1983. The costs for these services can't be included in the hospital's base year costs.

Uniform bill-payment summary (UB-82) System providing for the uniform collection of combined billing information and medical data.

Updating factor This is a percentage increase in the hospital market basket for goods and services plus 1 percent. The updating factor is applied to a hospital's base year costs for fiscal 1984 and 1985, after adjustment for budget neutrality.

Utilization management A multi-disciplinary hospital program for monitoring resource usage and quality of care.

Wage index The labor-related portion of a hospital's federal payment rates are multiplied by an urban or rural wage index that represents local hospital wages. The wage index varies depending on the metropolitan statistical area within which a hospital is located. Rural hospitals falling outside an MSA have a single wage index; this index varies by state.

Appendix C
SIMPLE PATIENT INFORMATION TOOL TO EXPLAIN BILLING

You will receive two separate bills for your x-ray examination

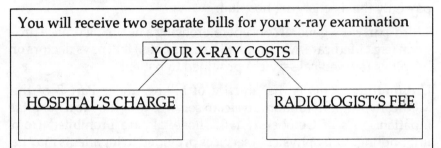

The hospital charge covers the cost of x-ray film, equipment, supplies and technical personnel.

The radiologist's fee covers the film interpretation which your doctor has requested.

4.11 QUALITY-ASSESSMENT AND IMPROVEMENT

Quality as a clearly defined and measurable objective has risen rapidly to the top of managers' agendas. Senior management is now touting quality as the essential ingredient for long-term success. Marilyn H. Sackett of Houston, Texas, reported the work of Philip B. Cosby on quality as follows:

> Quality is FREE; it is not a gift, but it is free. What costs money are all the actions that involve not doing the job right the first time. Quality can even be classified as an honest-to-goodness profit maker. Every penny saved on not doing things wrong or doing them over becomes a half a penny on the bottom line. In the current healthcare environment, where we do not know where our business will be tomorrow, there are very few ways left to improve our profit situation. If managers concentrate on making quality certain, we can probably increase the bottom line five to ten percent.

Sackett also states that the cost of quality is the expense of doing things wrong. Prevention is not hard to do; it is just hard to sell. Implementing a successful quality assessment and improvement program is impossible unless everyone in the department is involved. Training programs for employees play a major role in the effort. But quality improvement has no chance unless the individuals involved are ready to recognize that improvement is necessary. People perform to the standards of their leaders; if management thinks employees do not care, then they will not care.

In the healthcare industry, our main product is service to physicians and patients. They deserve to receive exactly what we have promised to produce. It is important to free ourselves of the myth that health care services cannot define what quality or outcome is for the marketplace. The current economic climate for health care has produced a survival race. Quality assessment and improvement programs are a good way to improve our services and reduce costs simply by doing the job right the first time.

According to Sackett, we must design programs and select monitors that will delineate those areas in operations that can be improved. Then we must educate our personnel about quality assessment and improvement and get them involved in implementation. Every employee must be trained to recognize the reasons for quality improvement and the results. Quality assessment and improvement then becomes the documentation of a job well done.*

The Challenge of the Quality Improvement Process in Radiology

The complexity of the quality assessment and improvement process in radiology is impacted by certain characteristics of practice that are unique to radiology. John Wilbanks and Kurt Mori, M.D., of Jacksonville, Florida, describe these special characteristics as follows:

- **Highly regulated:** "Radiology (with nuclear medicine and radiation oncology) has long been the most regulated specialty in medicine, largely because of its use of potentially harmful ionizing radiation." A key element of the quality management program relates to assuring the safety of patients and staff.
- **Hospital-based:** Hospital-based medical departments represent

---

* Sackett, M. H. "Quality Assurance Management: The Reasons and the Results." *Radiology Management*. 11(2) 1989: 54-55.

a hybrid in the quality management program because they must incorporate both administrative/technical components and professional components into the total process.

- **Marketer vs. gatekeeper tension:** There is tension between the administrator's role as marketer and promoter of the department's service capabilities and the role of gatekeeper who must assure tests referring physicians order are appropriate.
- **Single group:** Typically, all radiologists for a given hospital are members of a single group contracted to provide professional services. Quality issues that involve policing by one's own business associates can at times lead to a conflict of interests.
- **"Turf wars":** Quality management reviews of imaging interpretations and of interventional procedures performed in the radiology department typically are the responsibilities of the chief of radiology or a designee. With a growing trend of nonradiologist specialists entering the arenas of OB ultrasound, nuclear cardiology, prostatic ultrasound, and angiography, this responsibility is difficult because proposed credentialing and certification requirements and subsequent quality reviews can be seen as self-serving and protectionist.
- **Reading room review:** A unique feature of the interpretive facet of radiology is the daily review of the quality of one's work via "reading room" consultation with multiple specialists looking over the radiologist's shoulder.
- **Opportunities for correlation:** Given the proper information processing capabilities, diagnostic interpretation can be verified through correlation with pathologic, endoscopic, and surgical findings.
- **High volume, broad scope:** The volume and variety of work (interpretive and procedural) performed across all imaging modalities require the prudent use of sampling techniques that will validate quality management findings.
- **Third-party scrutiny:** Radiological procedures are being intensely scrutinized by third-party payers. Outpatient utilization review has already begun and clinical indications for studies are a prerequisite to payment for both inpatients and outpatients.*

---

* Wilbanks, J. and Kurt Mori. "Quality Management: Radiology's Challenge." *Administrative Radiology.* 9(10)1990:50-4.

The JCAHO's Ten-Step Process

According to the JCAHO, the quality assessment and improvement process involves the following:

- Identification of the most important aspects of care (e.g., procedures or treatments) provided by the organization, department, or service.
- Use of measurable indicators to systematically monitor these aspects of care in an ongoing way.
- Evaluation of care when thresholds are reached in the monitoring process, to identify problems in, or opportunities to improve, the quality and appropriateness of care.
- Taking actions to solve problems or improve the care and evaluation of the effectiveness of those actions.

Because the use of indicators to monitor important aspects of care involves the collection and aggregation of data about a series of events or activities, the monitoring and evaluation process can be used to identify trends or patterns of care that may not be evident when only case-by-case review is performed. Indicators can also be used to identify important single events that may represent poor quality care. Whether focused on patterns or single events, the use of indicators helps to identify situations efficiently in which case review (e.g., peer review) is most likely to identify correctable deficiencies in care or opportunities to improve care. Although the monitoring and evaluation process will not identify every case of substandard care, it does help the organization identify situations on which its attention could be most productively focused.

The ten step process provides a means for prioritizing quality improvement opportunities, analyzing findings, and reporting those findings in a way to suggest correction of deficiencies.

Step 1: Assign Responsibility

Each department director (or chairperson) should be responsible for, and actively participate in, monitoring and evaluation. The director assigns responsibility for the specific duties related to monitoring and evaluation. This responsibility is often delegated to the radiology manager.

Step 2: Delineate Scope of Care

Each department should consider the scope of care that it provides to establish a basis for identifying important aspects of care to monitor and evaluate. The scope of care is a complete inventory of what the department does. See Appendix A for a sample scope of care for radiology.

Step 3: Identify Important Aspects of Care

Important aspects of care are those that are high-risk, high-volume, and/or problem-prone. Staff should identify important aspects of care so monitoring and evaluation focuses on activities with the greatest impact on the quality of patient care.

Step 4: Identify Indicators

Indicators of quality should be identified for each important aspect of care. An indicator is a measurable variable related to a structure, process, or outcome of care. Examples of possible indicators (all of which would need to be further defined) include technologists who are not registered or do not possess equivalent experience (structure), preoperative chest x-rays not appropriate according to agreed-on protocol (process), and severe adverse reactions to contrast media (outcome).

Step 5: Establish Thresholds for Evaluation

A threshold for evaluation is the level or point at which intensive evaluation of care is triggered. Staff should agree on a threshold for each indicator. A threshold may be 0 percent or 100 percent or any other appropriate level. Setting a threshold at 0 percent or 100 percent means that the staff feels that even one occurrence in that area would be so serious or rare that it should trigger an intensive quality evaluation.

Step 6: Collect and Organize Data

Appropriate staff should collect data pertaining to the indicators. Data should be organized to facilitate comparison with the thresholds for evaluation.

Step 7: Evaluate Care

When the cumulative data related to an indicator reach the threshold for evaluation, appropriate staff members must evaluate the care provided to determine whether a problem exists. This evaluation, which may take the form of peer review, should focus on possible trends and performance patterns in addition to specific cases. The evaluation should also attempt to identify causes of any problems and methods by which care or performance may be improved.

Step 8: Take Actions to Solve Problems

When problems are identified, action plans must be developed, approved at appropriate levels, and enacted to solve the problem or take the opportunity to improve care.

Step 9: Assess Actions and Document Improvement

The effectiveness of any actions taken should be assessed and documented. If further actions are necessary to solve a problem, they should be taken and their effectiveness assessed.

Step 10: Communicate Relevant Information to the Organization-wide Quality Assessment and Improvement Program

Findings from and conclusions of monitoring and evaluation, including actions taken to solve problems and improve care, should be documented and reported monthly through the hospital's or imaging center's established channels of communication.*

When the JCAHO surveyor looks at the quality improvement program in radiology services, be prepared to answer these questions:

- What important aspects of care have been identified as relevant to your department/service/program?
- How were they chosen? Did department/service members participate in these determinations?

---

* *Examples of Monitoring and Evaluation in Diagnostic Radiology, Radiation Oncology and Nuclear Medicine Services.* Chicago: JCAHO, 1988.

- What indicators are in use in your department/service/program? Did department/service members participate in the identification of the indicators? Is each indicator relevant to activities in the department/service? Is each indicator a measurement of a relevant patient outcome or the measurement of a process that is believed to be related to patient outcomes? Is each indicator relevant to the staff involved in using it?
- How are the resulting data evaluated? Do department/service members participate in this evaluation, including the development of conclusions and recommendations?
- What has been done in response to the evaluation (e.g., what actions were taken)?
- How has the effectiveness of the action been evaluated?

The Quality Assessment and Improvement Plan (Example)

Anywhere Hospital
Diagnostic Imaging
Quality Assessment and Improvement Plan

In accordance with the hospital's Quality Assessment and Improvement Plan, the imaging center will monitor and evaluate major aspects of care.

RESPONSIBILITY

The Medical Director of the Center, with assistance from the Director, shall be responsible for implementing a planned and systematic process for monitoring and evaluating the quality and appropriateness of patient care rendered by each of the divisions of the Center for Diagnostic Imaging.

OBJECTIVES OF THE QUALITY ASSESSMENT AND IMPROVEMENT

1. To assure the implementation of an ongoing, planned, and systematic process to monitor and evaluate the care rendered to all patients served by the Center for Diagnostic Imaging.
2. To design a process that assures the important aspects of care of all the major clinical functions performed on all patient groups

served by the Center for Diagnostic Imaging are monitored and evaluated.

3. To aggregate data collected based upon objective criteria and indicators that are related to the quality and appropriateness of the important aspects of care rendered by all staff members of the Center for Diagnostic Imaging and that the staff members agree upon this objective methodology.

4. To implement a program that identifies problems as well as opportunities to improve the care provided by the Center for Diagnostic Imaging and take appropriate action to resolve the identified problems or to improve care.

5. To assure the continued effort of improving care and performance; to assess the effectiveness of actions taken; and to document the results. Results of all quality management activities are shared with members of the Center for Diagnostic Imaging quality management team.

6. To report conclusions and recommendations from the Center for Diagnostic Imaging monitoring and evaluation activities to the hospital-wide quality assessment program and to share, as appropriate, conclusions and recommendations with other departments and services.

SCOPE OF CARE

The scope of care of each of the divisions within the Center for Diagnostic Imaging is defined by its patient population, services, and setting. The scope of care in the Center for Diagnostic Imaging consists of a full service diagnostic imaging program.

IMPORTANT ASPECTS OF CARE

The Center for Diagnostic Imaging will annually review those aspects of care to assure that quality management reviews include high volume, high risk, and problem-prone areas.

INDICATORS

Indicators are specific to each aspect of care found in the Center for Diagnostic Imaging and may be identified separately. Examples of indicators would include appropriateness of examination, outcome, process, or the utilization of resources. These objective criteria will reflect current knowledge and clinical experience related to the important aspects of providing the care and services delivered by the Center for Diagnostic Imaging.

THRESHOLDS FOR EVALUATION

The thresholds for evaluation for the indicators in use in the Center for Diagnostic Imaging are determined by current clinical knowledge, national norms, and the historical experience of the department.

DATA COLLECTION/ANALYSIS

Concurrent and retrospective data collection is performed by appropriate personnel. Problems and opportunities to improve care will be identified from the information received from various data sources related to the aspects of care and any other information deemed as appropriate by the Director of the Center for Diagnostic Imaging. Data as it relates to the important aspects of care will be displayed and the resulting information evaluated to determine if an opportunity to improve care of a problem exists.

EVALUATION OF CARE

Findings from review activities and cases not meeting pre-established criteria are reviewed by the Director of the Center for Diagnostic Imaging. A preliminary review may be performed by other members of the department to identify and/or determine whether a problem exists, potential causes of problems identified and to evaluate possible trends and patterns of performance.

ACTION

Findings and problems that are identified in the review process are discussed at bi-weekly departmental meetings and action taken as appropriate by the director. Action alternatives may include but not be limited to policy development or revision, education, individual counseling, and performance evaluations.

ASSESSMENT AND DOCUMENTATION OF IMPROVEMENT

Once an opportunity to improve patient care is identified and action is taken, follow-up monitoring is conducted at appropriate intervals to assure continued problem resolution. Documentation of conclusions, actions, recommendations, and evaluation may be found in departmental minutes.

ORGANIZATIONAL COMMUNICATION AND INTEGRATION

Relevant information is communicated for further investigation/action/recommendation with other departments, committees, or individuals as considered appropriate. Summary reports from the Center for Diagnostic Imaging findings, conclusions, recommendations, actions taken and unresolved problems are forwarded to the institutional Quality Assessment and Improvement Committee.

STRUCTURE

There will be a quality assessment team in the Center for Diagnostic Imaging that will be utilized to evaluate the care rendered by the department. The members of this team will include the director, the medical directors of the various divisions, and the coordinators of each of the divisions of the Center for Diagnostic Imaging.

ANNUAL EVALUATION

On an annual basis, the Center for Diagnostic Imaging will evaluate its quality management activities based upon its plan and objectives. An annual report will be submitted to the institutional Quality Assessment and Improvement Committee for review. This evaluation will include a listing of all aspects of care reviewed during the year and a summary of those reviews and the results as to how patient care was improved.

Suggested Aspects of Care and Indicators to Monitor That Care

Kay Baker of Marietta, Georgia, has been collecting information for radiology managers to help in preparations for JCAHO visits and presenting that information each summer at the annual meeting of the American Healthcare Radiology Administrators. The following examples of important aspects of care and indicators to monitor that care are adapted from Baker's presentations.

Aspect of Care: Those procedures most frequently requested will be reviewed for appropriateness of utilization.
Indicators:

- Volume of CT of the head.
- Volume of chest x-rays.
- Ultrasound for pregnancy.

- Volume of portable examinations.
- Incidence of STAT requests.

Aspect of Care: Radiologic procedures with significant risk to the patient will be carefully monitored.
Indicators:

- Initial interpretations by emergency room physicians.
- Invasive procedures such as angiography and biopsies.
- Studies involving the use of contrast media.
- Radiologist's interpretations of mammography, chest radiographs for lung lesions.

Aspect of Care: Previously identified problem-prone areas in radiology services will be continuously monitored.
Indicators:

- Patient preparations.
- Utilization of portable services.
- Quality of portable radiographs.
- Timely reporting of results.
- Incidence of film retakes.
- Appropriateness of procedures ordered.
- Proper exam sequences.
- Availability of clinical indicators for the examination requested.
- Procedures for pediatric, geriatric and emergency patients.

Indicator Development

Indicators should correlate to important aspects of care identified in the radiology service menu. A threshold for evaluation should be assigned to each indicator monitored. The threshold establishes a rate beyond which intensive evaluation is expected. Thresholds may be adjusted, based on continuous monitoring data and evaluation of findings over a period of time. For example, the percentage of false-positive radiology diagnosis for cancer of the breast identified with mammography might be 15 percent. Or, the incidence of misadministrations of contrast media might be set at 0 percent.

A major responsibility for the radiology manager is to define the critical factors for measuring clinical performance. Lois Bittle of

Baltimore, Maryland, suggests that radiology departments look at measurable indicators of quality in the following service areas:

1. Aspiration during upper GI series.
2. Pneumothorax secondary to lung biopsy.
3. Contrast dye reactions.
4. Renal failure secondary to contrast dye reaction.
5. Cardiorespiratory arrests.
6. Repeat procedures due to inadequate preparation, inappropriate positioning, inappropriate exposure setting, equipment failure, inappropriate sequence, etc.
7. Radiologic findings that differ from surgical findings, pathology reports, clinical diagnosis.
8. Patients with first diagnosis of cancer who were x-rayed in the department in last six months.
9. Rereads with discrepancy in findings.
10. Patient complaints.
11. Patient satisfaction survey.
12. Procedure-specific arteriography/cardiac catheterization complications:
     - Arterial thrombosis, moderate hematoma, or circulatory compromise.
     - Seizures during or within 12 hours of procedure.
     - Extravasation of contrast material.
     - Metabolic problems.
     - Broken equipment, catheter, etc.
13. Postmyelogram arachnoiditis, seizure/convulsion, severe headache requiring narcotics.
14. Waiting times.
15. Lack of informed consent.
16. "Stat" requests.
17. X-ray requests without adequate clinical information.
18. Other incidents, (e.g., falls, IV infiltrates, rash, radiation burn secondary to overexposure).
19. Death within 24 hours of an invasive radiologic procedure.*

---

* McCue, Paul. "Consultant Services in Quality Assurance and Risk Management." *Applied Radiology*. 17(11)1988:23-4

Strategies to Meet Requirements

Given the current accreditation requirements and those yet to come as well as the desire to improve patient satisfaction and outcome, the following measures/recommendations should be considered by radiology managers.

1. Assess the strengths and weaknesses of the current quality assurance plan in the radiology department. A comprehensive plan should include four distinct formalized parts:
    *   quality control methods (machines, equipment, safety);
    *   traditional quality assurance screens for quality and risk;
    *   clinical criteria for quality care; and,
    *   process/systems review to promote improvement in patient care.

2. Revise the quality assurance plan to reflect the new changes and the method of implementation for CQI. This is necessary because:
    *   JCAHO requires an updated annual plan which should comply with new standards;
    *   aspects of care significant in improving patient outcomes need to be identified, as practice parameters may change; and,
    *   hospital governance must now be involved and appraised of quality activities in order to better guide the organization in policies impacting patient care.

3. Inform the medical staff of the results of quality improvement activities. The medical staff need to know how quality activities impact patient outcomes so they can examine the facts and make recommendations on policies surrounding the best measures to ensure the most appropriate care.

4. Establish processes to ensure that functional department supervisors are trained in the essence and importance of CQI. Radiology staff need to have fundamental knowledge in order to identify processes which could be improved in relation to patient care. Staff need to think in terms of the patient's perception of care.

5. Make certain that mechanisms are in place within each functional area in radiology to identify issues in relation to processes/systems

which can impact patient care. This can be done, for example, by staff referral to the CQI coordinator for inclusion of issues to be put on the agenda for review at the next meeting.

6. Determine how many man hours and additional costs are needed to comply with accreditation thrusts for the new process improvement. Sometimes, costs will increase in order to improve patient care processes to the outcome levels expected by the JCAHO.

7. Involve the functional departmental supervisors in assessing levels of patient satisfaction. This can be done through a variety of means, such as relaying the results of patient satisfaction surveys or registered patient complaints or compliments to the supervisors.

8. Encourage department staff to contribute ideas for innovative approaches to improving the patient perception of quality care. For example, a staff member may suggest erecting a sign with a 'panic button' so that when patients are experiencing undue delays or unsatisfactory service, they press the button for immediate management response.*

Conclusion

Everyone in your organization is taking the task of quality improvement and assessment very seriously. Assessing quality is an essential governance responsibility; your trustees will insist that an effective quality management program is in place and functioning and the "board" will be actively involved in evaluating the results of that program. The board of your organization will be asking if significant issues are being identified, if appropriate actions are being taken to correct problems, and if current practices meet regulatory requirements. Monroe E. Trout, M. D. and Jack A. Bernard of American Healthcare Systems, San Diego, California, suggest that corporate trustees are interested in reducing company liability. These are the typical issues that trustees want to be aware of:

• Problems that result in potentially compensable events, claims, or lawsuits.

---

* Bonnis, N., Micheletti, J., and Shlala, T. CQI Initiatives: Impact on Radiology. *Administrative Radiology*. 12(10):24. 1992.

- Problems that require disciplinary action by management or the medical staff executive committee.
- Problems that remain unresolved within a specific time frame.
- Management problems that require major capital expenditures:
  —Recurring patient complaints.
  —Problems that hurt public relations.

Trout and Bernard suggest that "integrity is the bottom line." On quality in healthcare, they describe the current quality assessment and improvement environment as a new and formidable challenge. Any organization has a tendency to react in such a way as to overcome a specific obstacle. Shrinking margins and diminishing access to capital represent the real challenge for hospitals. However, it is essential that when undertaking measures to improve the economic picture that we do not forget the basic mission: the delivery of high-quality care. If measurable quality becomes the focus, integrity of service to the patient and the community will be maintained and long-term success will be assured.*

Appendix A—Sample Scope of Care for a Diagnostic Radiology Department**

The department/service offers radiology services 24 hours per day to inpatients and emergency services patients of all ages. Range of treatments comprises diagnostic and therapeutic procedures, invasive/intraoperative and noninvasive techniques, and modalities using ionizing and (as in ultrasound) nonionizing radiation, with or without the use of contrast media.

Services including CT scanning, diagnostic ultrasound, and magnetic resonance imaging; and x-ray procedures constitute the majority of

---

* Trout, M.E. and J. A. Bernard. "Integrity is the Real Bottom Line." *Trustee*. 11. December 1988).
** Adapted from: *Examples of Monitoring and Evaluation in Diagnostic Radiology, Radiation Oncology and Nuclear Medicine Services*. Chicago: JCAHO, 1988.

the daily procedural load. Services related or concomitant to imaging include continuous quality assessment and improvement monitoring and evaluation, quality control, image interpretation, dictation, transcription, record filing/management, patient billing, marketing, equipment purchasing, film processing, and continuing education.

All individuals providing diagnostic radiology services and/or therapeutic radiation without supervision or direction have appropriate delineated clinical privileges. All individuals who provide technical diagnostic or therapeutic radiology services are licensed or registered and have the appropriate training and competence. Practitioners and staff include a physician director (board-certified radiologist), five other board certified radiologists (three with specialities in specific procedures or modalities, 30 registered technologists, a business manager, a hospital radiology manager, a darkroom technologist, secretarial/scheduling personnel, transcribers, consultants (radiation physicist and biomedical engineer), transportation aides, and registered nurses to respond to patient care needs before and during radiology procedures. During night shifts, technologists and radiologists are available by telephone or pager and able to respond in 30 minutes or less.

Technologists or other nonphysician personnel do not perform interventional studies or diagnostic fluoroscopy without a radiologist present, although the medical director may approve a trained nonphysician performing positioning procedure such as for cholecystograms.

Portable x-ray equipment allows radiographs to be obtained in surgery, as well as medical/surgical and intensive care units. Magnetic resonance imaging is permitted outside the institution by a mobile service.

Radiologists are consultants, and they are responsible for advising the referring physicians on which imaging procedures to perform. In addition, when emergency physicians request films and interpret them, staff radiologists are responsible for confirming or amending emergency physicians' initial interpretations.

Appendix B—Quality Assessment and Improvement Monitoring and Evaluation Form

Department: _____Radiology_____

Date Formulated: _____

Date Reviewed: _____

Aspects of Care:

Objective/Rationale:

Indicators: Threshold:

Methodology:

Data Sources:

Appendix C—Quality Assessment and Improvement Problem Tracking Sheet

Problem Identified	How Identified	Date Identified	To Whom Reported	Proposed Resolution	How Will Proposed Resolution Improve Pt Care?	Follow Up

Appendix D

Attach additional sheet if necessary.

Department _____

Quality Assessment Monitoring Criteria

Quarter Periods _____, _____, _____, _____

Summary of Indicator with Goal Statement	Threshold	Quarter	YTD	Quarter	YTD	Quarter	YTD	Quarter	YTD	Narrative Summary of Actual Performance

Appendix E—Glossary of CQI Terms*

Appropriateness of care The degree to which the correct care is provided, given current state-of-the-art knowledge; a component of quality of care.

Case mix The relative frequency of different diagnoses or conditions among patients.

Charge Statement of purpose given to a group of experts convened to develop a set of function-specific indicators during the indicator developmental process.

Comorbidity Disease or condition present at the same time as the principal disease or condition of a patient.

Continuity of care The degree to which the care needed by the patient is coordinated among practitioners and across organizations and time; a component of quality of care.

Continuous quality improvement An approach to quality management that builds upon traditional quality assurance methods by emphasizing the organization and systems (rather than individuals), the need for objective data with which to analyze and improve processes, and the ideal that systems and performance can always improve even when high standards appear to have been met; also called total quality management.

Data base An organized comprehensive collection of data.

Data element A single piece of information required by an indicator, subsequently aggregated in a manner with other data elements (i.e., indicator data collection logic) to identify indicator event occurences.

Data trend The general direction of indicator rates over time that may trigger further investigation of the event monitored by an indicator.

Effectiveness of care The degree to which care is provided in the correct manner; that is, without error, given the current state of the art; a component of quality of care.

---

*Adapted from: *Primer on Indicator Development and Application: Measuring Quality in Health Care.* JCAHO, 1990.

Efficacy of care   The degree to which a service has the potential to meet the need for which it is used; a component of quality of care.

Efficiency of care   The degree to which the care received has the desired effect with a minimum of effort, expense, or waste; a component of quality of care.

Expert   Individual who has knowledge and experience pertinent to a specified function.

Function   Goal-directed interrelated series of processes; some functions affect patients directly (e.g., most clinical processes) and others only indirectly (e.g., management processes and determining practitioner competence).

Health care organization   Health facility with organized staff that provides health-related services.

High-risk function   A key function that exposes individual patients to a greater chance of adverse occurrences if not carried out effectively and/or appropriately; also applies to services that are inherently risky, even when effective and appropriate, because of certain patient attributes and/or newness of the service.

High-volume function   A key function that is performed frequently or affects large numbers of patients. (e.g., diagnostic testing).

Indication   Guideline that specifies when certain course(s) of action are appropriate (e.g., for a specific disease or condition).

Indicator   Measurement tool used to monitor and evaluate the quality of important governance, management, clinical and support functions.

Indicator rationale   Indicator information set component that explains why an indicator is useful in specifying and assessing the process or outcome of care measured by the indicator.

Indicator statement   Indicator information set component that describes the function, activity, or event being assessed. (e.g., "patients for whom percutaneous transluminal coronary angioplasty has failed").

Key function   Goal-directed interrelated series of processes (e.g., function) that is believed (based on evidence or, at least, expert consensus) to have a significant effect on the probability of desired patient outcomes.

Mean   A measure of central tendency of data, for example, the sum of individual hospital indicator rates divided by the total number of hospitals contributing to a data base.

Medical record review   Process of reviewing patients' medical records to determine the existence of important quality-of-care questions relating to practitioner and/or organization factors.

Organization unit   A functional division of an organization.

Outcome   The result(s) of the performance (or nonperformance) of a function.

Process indicator   An indicator that measures an important discrete activity that contributes directly or indirectly to patient care; the best process indicators focus on processes that are closely linked to patient outcomes, meaning that a scientific basis exists for believing that the process, when provided effectively, will increase the probability of a desired outcome.

Provider   Healthcare professional or hospital, or a group of healthcare professionals or hospitals, that provide healthcare services to patients.

Quality of patient care   The degree to which patient care services increase the probability of desired patient outcomes and reduce the probability of undesired outcomes, given the current state of knowledge; determined by nine components: accessibility of care, appropriateness of care, continuity of care, effectiveness of care, efficacy of care, efficiency of care, patient perspectives issues, safety of the care environment, and timeliness of care.

Reliability assessment   The process of quantifying the accuracy with which indicator occurrences are identified from among all cases at risk of being indicator occurrences.

Scope of care   Inventory of processes that make up a specific function selected for indicator development; may include activities performed by governance, managerial, clinical and/or support staff personnel.

Sentinel event   A serious patient care event that requires further investigation each and every time it occurs; usually an undesirable, but may be a desirable, event.

Standard   Statement of expectation that defines organizations' structural and functional capacity to provide quality care.

Standards-based quality-of-care evaluation   Evaluation approach to quality of care that measures health care organizations' compliance with pre-established structure and process standards.

Threshold   The level at which a stimulus is strong enough to signal the need for organization response to indicator data and the beginning of the process of determining why the threshold has been crossed.

Timeliness of care   The degree to which care is provided to patients when it is needed; a component of care.

Validity assessment   The process of quantifying the extent to which indicators identify events that merit further review.

LIST OF REFERENCES—VOLUME 1

Abele, J. E. New tools extend value of intravascular therapy. *Diagnostic Imaging*. 12(9):57-63, 1990.

Abrams, H. L. Diagnostic technologies: the increasing role of technology assessment. *Decisions in Imaging Economics*. 3(2):29-34, 1990.

Ackerman, L. Digital storage of images. *Administrative Radiology*. 10(3):43-48, 1991.

Adams, H. G. Technologists staffing at the National Naval Medical Center. *Administrative Radiology*. 10(3):23-27, 1991.

"Advancement Programs in the Workplace." Summit on Manpower. Sudbury, MA. May, 1992, p. 3, 4, 6, 9, 23.

American College of Radiology Committee on Quality Assurance in Mammography, "Mammography Quality Control guidelines."

American College of Radiology, "Medicare Mammography Facility Checklist " Reston VA. March 1993.

American Hospital Publishing and the Linc Group, Inc. Profitable Healthcare Equipment. 1990.

Appleby, C. R. Cool laser won't replace balloon angioplasty. *Health Week*. 4(17):31, 1990.

Appleby, C. R. PET imaging: the elite technology. *Health Week*. 4(17):27-30, 1990.

Appleby, C. R. Running out: a scarcity of radiologic technologists, etc. *Health Week*. January 8, 1990.

Appleby, C. R. Suiting up with PACS. *Health Week*. 4(11): 29-32, 1990.

Aribisala, E.B. Applying the Americans with Disabilities Act to Radiology. *Radiology Management*. 15(2):27, 1993.

Bell, B. Careful strategy necessary for counselling effectively. *South Carolina Business Journal*. December 1987.

Berger, S. and Sudman, S.K. Physician/Hospital Trends for the 1990s Raise Some Red Flags. Healthcare Executive MAR/APRIL, 1992, P. 15.

Berkowitz, D. A. Managing your high-tech future. *Health Care Forum Journal*. 32(5):14-20, 1989.

Bittell, L.R. *What Every Supervisor Should Know*. N.Y.: McGraw Hill Book Company, 1980.

Black, W. C. MSI ferrets out electrical activity, identifies origins. *Diagnostic Imaging*. 13(1):74-76, 1991.

Boehme, J. and Choplin, R. RIS selection criteria part 2. *Administrative Radiology*. 9(10):69-71, 1990.

Bouchard, E. A. A business with a heart. *Continuing Care.* 9(3):22, 1990.

Bouchard, E. A. Consumer relations: another change for human resources. *Radiology Management.* 10(2):32, 1988.

Bouchard, E. A. Focused communication and physician bonding strategies. *Radiology Management.* 11(2):50-51, 1989.

Bowden, A. B. Negotiating a system purchase: 8 principles for protecting your institution's interest. *Health Care Executive.* 7(1):17-19, 1992.

Brice, J. Barriers begin to fall in bone densitometry. *Diagnostic Imaging.* 13(7):63-64, 1991.

Brightbill, T. Disk-contentment? *Health Week.* 4(18):21-25, 1990.

Brink, J. V. IMACS support shift toward enhanced service. *Diagnostic Imaging.* 13(9): 11-16, 1991.

Brotman, J. Breaking down barriers to customer focus. *Entrepreneur.* September 1989:14-16.

Bucci, R. Positron Emission Tomography: Executive Update Administrative Radiology. 12(5):53, 1993.

"Buyers' Guide to Evaluating MR Systems." GE Medical Systems. 1986.

Cannavo, M. J. Fitting PACS technology into the hospital of tomorrow. *Diagnostic Imaging.* 10(11):188-190, 1988.

Cannavo, M. J. Radiology information systems can improve department efficiency. *Diagnostic Radiology.* 10(12):92-95, 1988.

Cannavo, M. J. Small imaging companies capture IMACS market. *Diagnostic Imaging.* 13(9):31-34, 1991.

Cerne, F. Computer tomography alive and well. *Hospitals.* 62(27):65-69, 1988.

Cerne, F. Managing radiology data. *Hospitals.* 62(27):78-81, 1988.

Choplin, R. and Boehme, J. RIS the basics part 1. *Administrative Radiology.* 9(9):35-37, 1990.

"Choosing a Clinical Information System." Hewlett-Packard Company, 1990.

"Clinical Applications of Lasers." Laser Centers of America, 1989.

Coleman, E. PET: clinical positron emission tomography. *Administrative Radiology.* 9(6):34-41, 1990.

Courson, P. "On the Road: Planning and Operating a Mobile Mammography Program." *Administrative Radiology.* 10(4):48-58, 1991.

Cunningham, J. Make your next professional interview a success. *Administrative Radiology.* 9(12):25-28, 1990.

Curran, C. Telling it Like it is: Consultants Speak Out. *Second Source Imaging.* 8(3):52, 1993.

D'Agincourt, L. Lack of reimbursement impedes PET's growth. *Diagnostic Imaging.* 14(2):39-48, 1992.

D'Agincourt, Lori. PET's metabolic potency wins it clinical respect. *Diagnostic Imaging.* 14(1):68-75, 1992.

Davis, D., et al. "Meeting the Challenge—A Multidisciplinary Clinical Ladder Program." *Administrative Radiology.* 10:1 (16-20)91.

DeRosier, D. Using statistics to get the staff you need. *RT Image.* 3(37):1, 4-5, 18-19, 1990.

Dohms, J. *Hazard Communication Guidelines for Compliance,* " Sample Hazard Communication Program." *Radiology Management,* Fall 1992.

Dowd, S. Planning for the radiographer of the future. *Administrative Radiology.* 11(3): 36-43, 1992.

Doyle, E. T. Touring the mind with MSI. *RT Image.* 4(12):1, 4-6, 1991.

Eklund, G. W. and Brenner, R. J. The self-referred patient: a challenge to breast imaging practices. *Administrative Radiology.* 9(11):133-136, 1990.

Ellis, J. Employment Provisions in the ADA Protect Disabled from Discrimination. JMA Notes. Feb. 26, 1993, p. 1.

Eubanks, Paula. Hospitals struggle to respond to the technologist shortage. *Hospitals.* 64(14):32-37, 1990.

Fodor, J. Major equipment purchases: a committee approach. *Health Progress.* 69(10):12-14, 1988.

Friedman, G. Overcoming mammography phobia. *Health Week.* 4(7):19-23, 1990.

Gertman, P. M. Cost-containment measures radiology must respond. *Decisions in Imaging Economics.* 3(2):12-14, 1990.

Good, W. F., et al. PACS in radiology: a perspective. *Decisions in Imaging Economics.* 3(4):27-29, 1990.

Graham, J. Filmless radiology departments: fact or fiction. *Decisions in Technology Economics.* 1(1):11-15, 1988.

Greinacher, C. PACS: the patient care picture goes digital. *Seimens Review.* (4) 1988 pp. 3-7.

Gunther, R. Patient outreach: the key role of mammographic technologists in mammogram compliance. *Administrative Radiology.* 10(3):35-40, 1991.

Hall, L. T. Cardiovascular lasers: a look into the future. *American Journal of Nursing.* 90(7):27-30, 1990.

Hanlon, P. I. and Kaskiw, E. A. Physician bonding: one hospital's experience. *Computers in Healthcare.* 10(3):24-26, 1989.

Hanwell, L. The manpower shortage: it's everybody's problem. *Administrative Radiology.* 11(1):35-41, 1992.

Hatfield, S. PET technology advances into clinical settings. *Advance.* 2(8):1-4, 1989.

Hayden, L. and Nilges, E. Digital radiography with phosphur plates. *Administrative Radiology.* 10(5):44-47, 1991.

Hendee, W. R. Evolution of imaging far from complete. *Diagnostic Imaging.* 13(1):13-21, 1991.

Hendee, W. R. Radiology and physics: prognosis for the future. *Decisions in Imaging Economics.* 1(1):8-12, 1988.

Hendee, W. R. Transforming medical imaging from a craft into a science. *Diagnostic Imaging.* 10(11):97-103, 1988.

Henthorne, B. H. Look up from the book. *Administrative Radiology.* 9(10):47-48, 1990.

Hersey, P. and Blanchard, K. Management of Organizational Behavior. Englewood Cliffs, N.J., Prentice-Hall, Inc. 1982, pp. 41, 42.

Hess, T. P. Complexity of radiology management calls for computerized solutions. *Diagnostic Imaging.* 10(5):69-79, 1988.

Heuerman, J. N. Advice from a Head Hunter. *Healthcare Forum Journal.* 32(4):34-38, 1989.

Hopkins, E. M. A G.R.E.A.T. idea. *Health Progress.* 70(6):82-84, 1989.

Hoppszallern, S. and Handmaker, H. A national PET utilization forecast. *Administrative Radiology.* 11(2):32-37, 1992.

Huang, H. K. Implementing PACS: experience in future plans. *Decisions in Imaging Economics.* 3(2):20-24, 1990.

Hunter, D. P. and Jerew, M. Physician relationships in troubled hospitals. *Hospital Management Review.* 9(10):1, 1990.

Hunter, T. B. The personal computer in the radiologist's office. *Applied Radiology.* 20(8):33-36, 1991.

Institute for Clinical PET. 1991. "Average cost of a clinical PET scan based on procedures at 26 facilities."

Jaffe, C. C. and Lemke, H. U. Computer options open new radiology windows. *Diagnostic Imaging.* 13(9):21-28, 1991.

JCAHO Recommended Plant/Safety Orientation. *New Employee Orientation.*

Johnson, D. Relationship management clearly differentiates hospitals. *Healthcare Strategic Management.* 7(8):2-3, 1989.

Jones, W. J. Letting technology dictate design. *Healthcare Strategic Management.* 6(11):10-12, 1988.

Katzen, B. T. Lasers and other vascular devices may augment balloon angioplasty. *Diagnostic Imaging.* 10(4):55-56, 1988.

Ketchum, L. E. RSNA 1991: technical highlights. *Applied Radiology.* 21(1):62-70, 1992.

King, G. R. Let the employer beware. *Modern Healthcare's Facilities Operation and Management.* 21(18):24-25,1991.

Krug, H. Subsidizing screening mammography through induced revenues and profits. *Radiology Management.* 12(4):28-32, 1990.

Kuber, M. S. Radiologic administration: structure and style. *Radiology Management.* 2(1):6-15, 1980.

Kurzweil Applied Intelligence, Inc. Voice Recognition Generated Report. Walttham, MA.

Langley, M. ADA Expected to change jobs, hiring. The Knoxville News Sentinel, June 27, 1993.

Lester, B. *Verifying references.* Johnstown, PA.

Lester, B. *What You Can and Can't Ask During an Interview.* Johnstown, PA.

Levine, B. and Bozarth, C. A guide to PACS-RIS/HIS communication. *Administrative Radiology.* 11(1):43-47, 1992.

Linn, B. Hospital use lags behind laser's tremendous potential. *Healthcare Strategic Management.* 7(8):1, 19-23,1989.

Lumsdon, K. Moving target: hospitals take careful steps in acquiring PET. *Hospitals.* 66(7):58-62, 1992.

Lynch, Maureen. Department directors provide the steps to heavenly imaging. *Administrative Radiology.* 11(3):51-53, 1992.

Mace, J. Approaching clinical advancement in radiology. *Radiology Management.* 13(4):45, 1991.

"Magnetic Resonance Imagers." *Healthweek.* November, 1990.

Maner, P. and Hamilton, T. The team approach. *Administrative Radiology.* 11(2):39-43, 1992.

"Manpower Networking Resource." *Summit on Manpower.* 1990.

Mayer, J. Find the Job You've Always Wanted in Half the Time and with Half the Effort (1992) Contemporary Books. Adapted by *The Pryor Report* Vol 9(1):9, 1993.

McCue, P. The shortage of radiologic technologists. *Applied Radiology.* 19(5):28-31, 1989.

Melbin, J. E. Challenging the gold standard. *RT Image.* 5(3):4-9, 1992.

Melbin, J. E. Hyperthermia: the fourth frontier. *RT Image.* 9(29):1, 4-6, 35, 1991.

Meyer, P., et al. The American College of Radiology Mammography Accreditation Program. *Administrative Radiology.* 9(8):28-36, 1990.

Mitigui, J. The waiting room. *Health Progress.* 68(1):122, 1987.

Nabi, H. A. Antibody imaging in colon cancer. *Applied Radiology.* 21(2):59-64, 1992.

Nelson, M. The shortage of radiologic technologists. *Decisions in Imaging Economics.* 2(1):20-25, 1990.

News Briefs: Bush signs mammography bill. *Second Source Imaging.* 8(1):14,1993.

New Britain MRI. Sample floor plan of MRI facility. New Britain, Conn.

Nielsen, G. A. How to make salary comparisons and negotiate a raise. *Radiology Management.* 13(1):52-3, 1991.

Nowak, S. Patient power: a commentary. *Administrative Radiology.* 11(2):55, 1992.

O'Leary, T. J., et al. Screening mammography: barriers and incentives. *Applied Radiology.* 20(9):11-17, 1991.

"PACS: A NEMA Primer." The National Electrical Manufacturers Association, 1988.

"PACS Components." *Healthweek.* June 11, 1990.

"PACS in Place in the United States." *Diagnostic Imaging:* Focus on PACS. September, 1990.

Parker, M. A. Risk of malpractice escalates in breast cancer screening. *Diagnostic Imaging.* 10(7):82-85, 1988.

Peterson, K. Caring for people, not profits, brings success. *Modern Healthcare.* 20(39):34, 1990.

Powills, S. Mobile technology takes radiology on the road. *Hospitals.* 62(21):80, 1988.

Press, I. and Gainey, R. What experiences contribute to satisfaction with the hospital? *Michigan Hospitals.* September 1990, pp. 17-21.

Rooney, M. Resume rules for healthcare executives. *Healthcare Executive.* 6(4):35, 1991.

Rowe, W. M. Upgrading a radiology information system. *Radiology Management.* 12(2):24-28, 1990.

Rowe, W. Purchase considerations for a radiology information system. *Radiology Management.* 14(1):43-45, 1992.

Ryan, K. and Oestreich, D. *Driving Fear Out of the Workplace,* Jossey-Bass: San Francisco, CA. Adapted by *The Pryor Report,* Vol 19(1):8, 1993.

Schmitz, S., et al. The current status of bone densitometry. *Applied Radiology.* 19(6):20-26, 1990.

Schwartz, H. W. Evaluating productivity and budgeting staff. *Radiology Management.* 11(3):39, 1989.

Schwartz, H. W. Practical considerations in evaluating a radiology information management system for your environment. *Radiology Management.* 13(3):30-35, 1991.

Schwartz, H.W. "Justifying Capital Equipment in the 1990's." *Radiology Management.* 12(2):35-39, 1990.

Seago, K. Scoring a radiology department's niceness factor. *Applied Radiology.* 15(1):49-51, 1986.

Seshadri, S. B. Mini-PACS help solve image problems today. *Diagnostic Imaging.* 13(9):17-19, 1991.

Siemens/CTI PET Systems Nuclear PET Group. Knoxville, TN.

Skillington, C.J. "Directory of Technologist Education in MRI." *R.T. Image Magazine.* Oct. 26, 1992.

Skjei, E. UCLA tackles obstacles to filmless department. *Diagnostic Imaging.* 13(9):3-9, 1991.

Solomon, A. and Martino, S. Relative value units: practical productivity management. *Radiology Management.* 13(1):33-35, 1991.

Southwick, K. MABS: the imaging phenom. *Health Week.* 4(22):62-64, 1990.

Stockburger, W. T. and King, W. E. PACS: a financial analysis for economic viability. *Applied Radiology.* 19(1):17-24, 1990.

Straub, W. H. and Dey, A. A. So you want to get into the breast imaging business? *Administrative Radiology.* 8(7):14-17, 1989.

"Summit on Manpower, Report: April 1989." Summit on Manpower.

"Tech shortage spurs Summit actions." *ACR Bulletin.* vol. 47(3), 1991.

"Technology on Wheels: Evaluating the Options." *Health Technology.* 1(6):231-238, 1987.

Tighe, L.C. PET: When Will it Get Here? *Second Source Imaging.* 7(12):40-2, 1992.

Tilke, B. Equipment purchases demand skill savvy—and specifics. *Advance.* 3(35): 1-9, 1990.

Tsuchiyama, S. Difficult questions: treating the self-referred patient. *Administrative Radiology.* 9(11):129-132, 1990.

Wachel, W. Do you know your physicians? *Healthcare Executive.* 7(2):14-17, 1992.

Wagner, M. "Keep Unique...for PET" *Modern Healthcare.* November 30, 1992.

Wagner, M. Establishing Pet Charges Requires Identification of Total Costs. *Modern Healthcare.* November 30, 1992. p. 38.

Wagner, M. Weighing the costs of new technology. *Modern Healthcare.* 18(34):43-58, 1988.

Walklett, W. and Green, J. Heat as a diagnostic aid. *Administrative Radiology.* 9(12):57-59, 1990.

Walt, A. J. Screening and breast cancer: a surgical perspective. *American College of Surgeons Bulletin.* 75(9):6-10, 1990.

Wedel, C.S. The Americans with Disabilities Act: The Impact on Radiologic Technologists and Managers. *Radiology Management,* 15(2):23, 1993.

Weinstein, A. Hospitals should say no to some technologies. *Hospitals.* 64(18):80, 1990.

Weiss, R. Appealing to an important customer. *Health Progress.* 70(4):38-45, 1989.

Wesolowski, C. E. Show that you care. *Radiology Management.* 12(4):34-38, 1990.

West, Michael G. Information system can save money while improving patient care. *Diagnostic Imaging.* 10(5):159-162, 1988.

Whelan, M.C. Getting to the Bone. *Second Source Imaging.* 7(4): 50-57, 1992.

Wood, C. J. How much does an employee really cost? *RT Image.* 3(43):1, 6, 7, 21, 1990.

Worth, J. Your crystal image: developing your resume. *Administrative Radiology.* 9(12):22-24, 1990.

LIST OF REFERENCES—VOLUME 2

"Administrator's Guide to MR." GE Medical Systems, 1990.

"A Layman's Guide to Hospitals: An Introduction to Finance and Economics." Coopers and Lybrand, 1978.

Albrecht, K. *Service Within*, Dow Jones-Irwin, Homewood, IL. As adapted by The Pryor Report Vol 9(1):9, 1993.

Anderson, H. J. Survey identifies trends in equipment acquisitions. *Hospitals.* 64(18):30, 32-35, 1990.

Annis, R . Budgeting: getting to the bottom line. *Health Progress.* December 1988, pp. 74-76.

Annis, R. Accounts receivable: how to monitor and control them. *Health Progress.* May 1988, pp. 70-71.

Appleby, C. R. Spreading the word: hospitals market imaging services by educating consumers, physicians. *Health Week.* 4(5):37-43, 1990.

Arbeiter, J. S. Are you merely a witness to the patient's consent? *RN* 51(10):53-57, 1988.

ARC Standard for Communication—Diagnostic Radiology. *ACR Bulletin.* 11/91.

Bartlett, E. E. Talk to your patients to avoid trouble later with malpractice. *Diagnostic Imaging.* 9(11):179-187, 1987.

Bergey, T. W. Sorting out the three r's: RVU, RVS and RBRVS. *Radiology Management.* 13(4):35-39, 1991.

Bogardus, C. Billing tactics: advantages of a professional billing service in radiation oncology. *Administrative Radiology.* 10(1):51-56, 1991.

Bonnis, N., Micheletti, J., and Shlala, T. CQI Initiatives: Impact on Radiology. *Administrative Radiology.* 12(10):24. 1992.

Bouchard, E. Service line management. *Radiology Management.* 14(1):22-23, 1992.

Bradley, L. Industry strategies have appropriate home in hospitals. *Healthcare Strategic Management.* 8(6):8-13, 1990.

Brice, J. "Simple Tactics Minimize Exposure to Malpractice." *Diagnostic Imaging.* 14(3):44-45, 1992.

Brice, J. CON regs loosen grip on imaging equipment. *Diagnostic Imaging.* 12(9):73-76, 1990.

Brown, S. W. and Morley, A. P. Marketing through the medical staff. *Healthcare Executive.* 1(2):45-48, 1986.

Brown, S.W. and Morley, A.P. *Marketing Strategies for Physicians.* Oradell, NJ, Medical Economics Books. 1986, p. 130.

Brumbaugh, J., et al. Conversion to nonionics packs economic punch. *Diagnostic Imaging.* 13(7):99-104, 1991.

Buff, H. "Preparing for the JCAH survey." *Administrative Radiology.* 6(7):28-32, 1987.

Burke, M. Chilling effect on mergers? *Trustee.* 43(8):20-21, 1990.

"Buyers Guide to Evaluating MR Systems." GE Medical Systems, 1986.

Byers, K. D. and Livingston, C. A framework for writing a business plan. Management Issues. Peat Marwick Main and Company, 1989.

Carswell, H. Older MRI systems yield $500,000± in profits. *Diagnostic Imaging.* 13(7):41-44, 1991.

Chapman-Cliburn, G. Risk management and quality assurance: issues and interactions. *Quality Review Bulletin.* 1986.

"Coaching and Counselling." Stewart and Associates, Inc., Columbia, SC, 1990.

Conley, D. J. and Greenberg, J. Financial considerations in purchasing technical equipment. *The Journal of Medical Practice Management.* 3(1):23-26, 1987.

"Creating a Winning Marketing Campaign." American Management Association, 1990.

Curran, C. Government regulations. *Second Source Imaging.* 7(3):32-38, 1992.

Dey, A. The ABC's of billing. *Administrative Radiology.* 9(4):39-41, 1990.

Di Giacinto, T. M., et al. The MRI decision process. *Administrative Radiology.* 9(1):27-30, 1990.

Dickes, L. *Reimbursement Lingo* from "Influencing Reimbursement." *RT Image.* 3(27): 16-17, 1990.

DiStefano, M. and Orlandi, A. V. Historical facts regarding limited licensure. *RT Image.* 3(40):5, 22, 1990.

Dowd, S. Planning for the radiographer of the future. *Administrative Radiology.* 11(3):36-43, 1992.

Doyle, E. T. The fight for licensure goes on. *RT Image.* 4(31):10-11, 36-37, 1991.

Drane, J. F. and Roth, R. B. Medical decision making for the incompetent patient. *Health Progress.* 68(12):37-42, 1987.

Drew, P. G. Walking the tightrope bridging cost and quality. *Diagnostic Imaging.* 13(7):57-60, 1991.

"Eleven Safe Harbors to Find." *ACR Bulletin.* 47(9):1, 4-11, 1991.

Eubanks, P. Acclamating the new exec should be first goal. *Hospitals.* 65(5):50, 1991.

Eubanks, P. Clinicians: manage your move to manager. *Hospitals.* 65(5):60, 1991.

Examples of Monitoring and Evaluation in Diagnostic Radiology, Radiation Oncology and Nuclear Medicine Services. Chicago: JCAHO, 1988.

Faden, A. I. and Faden, R. R. Informed consent in medical practice: with particular reference to neurology. *Archives of Neurology.* 35(11):761-764, 1978.

Fischer, H. W. Raising department efficiency with concentric zone design. *Diagnostic Imaging.* 10(9):168-170, 1988.

Fisk, T. A. The marketing matrix: adopting an analytic approach. *Decisions in Imaging Economics.* 2(4):12-19, 1989.

Gardner, E. UB-82 forms offer wealth of information, misinformation. *Modern Healthcare.* 20(38):18-29,1990.

Glossary of JCAHO Terms. *JCAHO Accreditation Manual for Hospitals.* 1992.

Goldsmith, M. and Leebov, W. Strengthening the hospital's marketing position through training. *Healthcare Management Review.* 11(2):83-93, 1986.

Green, A. M. RVS puts radiologists at forefront in medicine's search for values. *Diagnostic Imaging.* 11(6):63-66, 1989.

Greene, J. "A Strategy for Cutting Back: screening processes mark money–losing services for closing. *Modern Healthcare.* 19(33):29-47, 1989.

Gur, D., et al. A perspective of the resource-based relative value scale. *Administrative Radiology.* 10(3):28-34, 1991.

Hansen, R. F. Increasing market share through good design. *Healthcare Strategic Management.* 5(3):15-21, 1987.

Harms, S. Magnetic resonance imaging. *Administrative Radiology.* 9(8):39-49,1990.

Hatfield, S. Administrators look to build confidence in construction decisions. *Advance.* 4(32):24-25,1991.

Hatfield, S. RT's and the law: a few precautions can reduce risk of lawsuits. *Advance.* 2(10):14-15, 1989.

Hayward, J. 1992 CPT coding changes. *Administrative Radiology.* 11(3):45-47, 1992.

Healthweek—Desktop Resource. Healthcare Knowledge Systems (CPHA). September 24, 1990. Ann Arbor, MI.

Hess, T. P. Personal contact, not a hard sell, wins referrals for MRI services. *Diagnostic Imaging.* 10(3):67-72, 1988.

"History of the ARRT Involvement with State Licensure." ARRT Annual Report, 1989. p. 3.

Hoppszallern, S. MRI: a forecast for the future. *Administrative Radiology.* 9(8):51-55, 1990.

"How safe are your harbors?" *Imaging Economics.* Vol. 1, No. 1, March 1992. p. 7.

"How Should Stereotactic Breast Biopsy be Coded?" The RMBA Bulletin. November 1992. Costa Mesa, CA.

"How to Use CPT Coding." Medi-Index Publications. Salt Lake City, Utah. 6(3):3, 1991.

Hudson, T. Hospital/MD joint ventures move forward despite hurdles. *Hospitals.* 65(9):22-28, 1991.

Hughes, C. and Van Gilse, M. Tracking the elusive MRI referral pattern. *Administrative Radiology.* 9(11):111-114, 1990.

Hughes, C. Consider financial options prior to leasing equipment. *Diagnostic Imaging.* 11(8):40-41, 137, 1989.

Hughes, C.M. "MRI centers must sell themselves to survive in competitive market." *Diagnostic Imaging.* 10(7):95, 1988.

Hulley SB, Cummings SR, eds. *Designing Clinical Research: An Epidemiologic Approach.* Baltimore: Williams & Wilkins, 1988, p.43. Imaging Economics Newsletter. Vol, No. 4, 1993, p. 2.

Hunton, B. W. Good planning takes organization. *Advance.* 4(32):24-25, 1991.

Hunton, B.W. Protocols: Guide use of non-ionic contrast media. Advance for Administrators. 2(5):11, 1992.

Iglehart, J. K. and White, J. K. Hospital industry divided on Medicare capital payments. *Health Progress.* 68(1):17-18, 93, 1987.

"Improving Report Turnaround Time to Increase Referrals." *Imaging Market Forum.* 5(2):1-5, 1988.

"IRS Acts on Joint Ventures." *ACR Bulletin.* 48(2):1, 5-6, 1992.

Jablonski, J.R. Implementing Total Quality Management in the 1990's. Technical Management Consortium, Inc. Albuquerque, N.M., 1991, p. 81.

Johnson, G. Total quality management: will it work for me? *Radiology Management.* 14(1):30-31, 1992.

Johnson, K. C. MRI centers: ten design mistakes to avoid. *Hospitals.* 61(7):82-84, 1987.

Jones-Bey, H. Radiologists in quandary over ethics of nonionics. *Diagnostic Imaging.* 14(2):9-15, 1992.

Kanal, E. Taking a logical approach to MRI system acquisition. *Diagnostic Imaging.* 10(8):73-80, 182, 1988.

Katayama, H. The contrast media controversy: implications of a landmark safety study. *Administrative Radiology.* 9(9):20-22, 1990.

Keefe, J. and Sullivan, R. New planning assumptions needed in deregulated imaging climate. *Diagnostic Imaging.* 9(10):71-75, 1987.

Keenan, L. A. and Goldman, E. F. "Positive Imaging: Design as Marketing Tool in Diagnostic Centers." *Administrative Radiology.* 8(2):36-41, 1989.

Keenan, L. Design and architecture in radiology. *Administrative Radiology.* 9(6):43-48, 1990.

Kidd, K. L. Radiology reimbursement. *Applied Radiology.* 18(5):16-21, 1989.

Koska, M.T., JCAHO Introduces three new areas of survey concentration. *Hospitals.* Oct. 5, 1992, pp. 62-64.

Kropf, R. Developing a competitive advantage in the market for radiology services. *Hospital and Health Services Administration.* 33(2):213-220, 1988.

Kukla, S. F. *Cost Accounting and Financial Analysis for the Hospital Administrator.* American Hospital Publishing, Inc., 1986.

Kuntz, L. A. Medical negligence. *RT Image.* 5(1):4-5, 17, 1992.

Kyes, K. A Nationwide Review. *Decisions in Imaging Economics.* Vol. 5, No. 3, 1992.

Labovitz, G. H. Beyond the total quality management mystique. *Healthcare Executive.* 6(2):15-17, 1991.

Lawson, T. C. Joint ventures: a legal evaluation. *Decisions in Imaging Economics.* 3(3): 1990.

Leckie, R. et al. Surveying for Excellence in Radiology. *Administrative Radiology.* 12(8):34, 1992.

Leiter, P. and Jacobson, S. L. "Sound Marketing for Off Site Private Practices." *Rehab Management.* 4(6):37-40, 1990.

Lille, K. "Applying for a Certificate of Need." *Radiology/Nuclear Medicine Magazine.* 7(4):29, 1977.

Long, H. W. Cash flow, capital costs and provider incentives. *Decisions in Imaging Economics.* 3(4):22-26, 1990.

"Low Osmolality Contrast Media: Choice and Challenge for the '80's." Special Supplement. *Diagnostic Imaging.* 9(12):1-32, 1987.

Lucchese, D. R. and Eikman, E. A. The medical-legal implications of contrast agent use. *Applied Radiology.* 18(12):36-37, 1989.

Lynch, Maureen. Department directors provide the steps to heavenly imaging. *Administrative Radiology.* 11(3):51-53, 1992.

Lynch, R. "Reimbursement Management Primer for DRG and ICD-9 Analysis." *Journal of Cardiovascular Management.* 2(1):41-48, 1990.

"Magnetic Resonance Glossary." Siemens Medical Systems, Inc., 1988.

Maltzer, R. The hazards of outcome measures. *Administrative Radiology.* 11(1):51-52, 1992.

Maner, P. and Hamilton, T. The team approach. *Administrative Radiology.* 11(2):39-43, 1992.

"Market-based strategies boost imaging referrals." *Diagnostic Imaging.* 15(1):23, 1993.

"Marketing: A Four Step Process." *The Medical Network: Emergency and Convenience Care News.* September 1988, pp. 3-4.

Martin, J. Maslow and manpower: a humanistic approach to technologist retention. *RT Image.* 2(31):10-12, 1989.

Matson, Holleman, Nosek and Wilkinson. *The Journal of Family Practice.* 36(2): 204-205, 1993.

McAtte, J. A. Practical guidelines to responding to court subpeonas. *The Journal of Medical Practice Management.* 3(1):47-51, 1987.

McCue, P. "Consultant Services in Quality Assurance and Risk Management." *Applied Radiology.* 17(11):23-24, 1988.

McCue, P. Diagnostic imaging centers: turnkeys complete. *Applied Radiology.* 16(9): 27-34, 1987.

McIlrath, S. Bad news on RBRVS rules. *AMA News.* June 17, 1991, pp. 1, 28-29.

Meehan, C.H. "The Guide to Department Planning." Columbia, S.C.

Mescon, M. H. and Mescon, T. S. Leading by inspiration: an example. *Sky.* 20(4):102-104, 1991.

Mescon, M. H. and Mescon, T. S. One customer at a time. *Sky.* 20(2):100-101, 1991.

Miccio, J. A. The migration of medical technology. *Healthcare Forum Journal.* 32(5):23-26, 1989.

Michael, K. The evolution of continuing education in the field of allied health. *Administrative Radiology.* 11(1):27-28, 1992.

Morrison, J. Malpractice issues in the education of healthcare professionals, part 1. *Advance.* 2(14):1-3, 28, 1989.

Morrison, J. Malpractice issues in the education of healthcare professionals, part 2. *Advance.* 2(15):7-9, 1989.

Motyka, E. A step above: marketing the cancer center. *Administrative Radiology.* 9(9):51-52, 1990.

Musfeldt, C. The Last Word: 10 Attributes of a hassle-free hospital. *Hospitals.* August 20, 1992. p. 76.

Newbold, P. A. Emerging new relationships: from the customer's perspective. *Hospital Entrepreneur's Newsletter.* 3(1):4-7, 1987.

"Nonionic Contrast Media: Selective or 100% Usage?" Special Supplement. *Diagnostic Imaging.* 89(12):1-20, 1990.

Nowak, S. F. Living with the budget. *Applied Radiology.* 17(10):28, 77-78, 1989.

Nyberg, M. Turn around time: a financially troubled Philadelphia hospital goes out of the red and into the black. *Health Progress.* 72(7):57-61, 1991.

O'Dell, C. Building on received wisdom. *Healthcare Forum Journal.* 36(1): 17-8, 1993.

Olsen, G. G. Business venture restrictions. *Rehab Management.* 5(1):106-107, 1992.

"Organization Directory: 1992." *Administrative Radiology.* 11(1):55-61, 1992.

"Organizations in Radiology." American College of Radiology, 1990.

"Patient Satisfaction Survey." American Healthcare Radiology Administrators, 1993.

Placone, R. C. and Farr, M. H. Steering a center from startup to success. *Administrative Radiology.* 9(2):36-40, 1990.

Placone, R. C. The mid-field MRI center: 1990's answer to the continuing crisis in healthcare costs. *Administrative Radiology.* 9(10):55-62, 1990.

"Planning a new MRI Facility: Avoiding Common Mistakes." *Imaging Economics.* Vol. 1, No. 3, 1992.

"Potential Antitrust Violations." *ACR Bulletin.* 47(6):16-18, 1991.

"Preparing a Business Plan: A Guide for the Emerging Company." Ernst and Whinney, 1987.

Primer on Indicator Development and Application: Measuring Quality in Health Care. JCAHO, 1990.

"Principles for a Sound Quality Effort." *The Westrend Letter.* September 1990, p. 3.

"Professional Organizations." *1992 Radiology Reference Guide.* Access Publishing Co., pp. 161-164.

"Radiology Reimbursement Reference: To Guide You Through the Maze of Radiology Reimbursement." American Healthcare Radiology Administrators, 1990.

Reuter, S. R. An overview of informed consent for radiologists. *AJR.* 148:219-227, 1987.

Rollo, F. D. Patient protection: utilizing quality control measures for success. *Decisions in Imaging Economics.* 3(5):4-7, 1990.

Roper, R. R. How to loose informed consent. *Applied Radiology.* 18(4):8-10, 1989.

Rostenberg, B., Campbell, J., and Stein, M. "Managing Successful Radiology Projects." RSNA '92 presentation. Chicago, Ill.

Rudnick, J. D. A process and considerations for activating a quality/productivity monitoring system. *Healthcare Strategic Management.* 5(3):23-27, 1987.

Sackett, M. H. "Quality Assurance Management: the Reasons and Results." *Radiology Management.* 11(2)1989:54-55.

Schonfeld, A. R. Marketing radiology to referring physicians. *Applied Radiology.* 17(11):9, 1988.

Schonfeld, A. R. Teleradiology: examining its impact on imaging management. *Decisions in Imaging Economics.* 2(4):20-25, 1989.

Schwartz, H. W. Justifying capital equipment in the 1990's. *Radiology Management.* 12(2):35-39, 1990.

Schwartz, H. W. Managing radiology in the 1990's, part 1. *Applied Radiology.* 19(7):13-16, 1990.

Scott, C. and Jaffe, T. *Managing Organizational Change*, Crisp Publications. Los Altos, CA. As adapted by the Pryor Report Vol 9(1):6, 1993.

Seago, K. Imaging center design and construction: good planning pays off. *Applied Radiology.* 16(2):37-42, 1987.

Seaver, D. J. Taking charge: winning strategies for hospital CEOs in new positions. *Healthcare Executive.* 5(6):13-16, 1990.

"Self-referral Deplored." *ACR Bulletin.* 48(1):1, 4-5, 1992.

Shorr, A. S. Structuring and negotiating the deal. *Healthcare Strategic Management.* 5(8):4-7, 1987.

Simmons, J. E. Holding marketing accountable. *California Hospitals.* 2(4):18-21, 1988.

"Six Steps to Choosing the Right Corporate Consultant." *Hospitals.* 65(13):45, 1991.

Smith, P. A. Uncover the hidden technical component. *Update.* 6(3):1-5, 1991.

Solomon, M. A. Put emotions aside when assessing whether or not to open MRI center. *Diagnostic Imaging.* 10(11):163-169, 1988.

"Sound Planning and Design for Technology-Related Construction: The Ultimate High Technology." *Health Technology.* 1(6):247-254, 1987.

Spring, D. B. Radiologists approach concensus on informed consent procedures. *Diagnostic Imaging.* 10(11):171-172, 1988.

"Staff Gains Confidence in Total Quality Management Through Its Use in Effective Problem-Solving at 500-bed Medical Center Hospital of Vermont." *Healthcare Productivity Report.* 4(2):1-7, 1991.

"Starting and Managing Your Radiology Imaging Center." *Winthrop Pharmaceuticals—Diagnostic Imaging Division.*

Steel, J. and Perry, J. Reducing repeat films through a total quality Management Approach. *Administrative Radiology.* 11(2):47-49, 1992.

Stewart, D. Equipment leasing: a guide for lessees. *Administrative Radiology.* 9(2):87-90, 1990.

Stier, R. D. Creating an effective marketing team. *Healthcare Executive.* 4(3):36-38, 1987.

Stone, D. A. How to prepare a radiology policy and procedure manual. *Radiology Management.* 2(2):16-20, 1980.

"Strategic Planning Doesn't Stop With the Plan." *Optimal Health.* 3(4):25, 1987.

Straub, W. and Gur, D. Optimizing performance of the billing company. *Administrative Radiology.* 10(1):38-40, 1991.

Studnicki, J. Measuring service line competitive position: a systematic methodology for hospitals. *Health Progress.* 72(6):68-72, 1991.

Templeton, N. Procedural coding evolves. *ACR Bulletin.* 48(1):9-11, 1992.

Tilke, B. RT's continue to wage battle for licensure. *Advance.* 3(43):1-2, 9, 1988.

Tokarski, C. Revised Stark bill still packs enough wallop to slow ventures. *Modern Healthcare.* 19(29):34-36, 1989.

"Top 25 Most Frequently Performed Radiology Procedures." Healthcare Knowledge Systems (CPHA). Ann Arbor, MI. *Healthweek—Desktop Resource. September 24, 1990.*

Trout, M. E. and Bernard, J. A. "Integrity is the Real Bottom Line." *Trustee.* 41(12):11, 1988.

Tsuchiyama, S. How to build the perfect technologist. *Administrative Radiology.* 9(12):44-52, 1990.

Urban, C. D. Market-driven communication strategy. *The Healthcare Forum Journal.* 34(1):24-27, 50, 1991.

Wagner, M. Promoting hospital's high-tech equipment. *Modern Healthcare.* 18(47):43-48, 62-58, 1988.

Wagner, S. K. IRS policy raises another barrier to joint venturing. *Diagnostic Imaging.* 14(2):24, 1992.

Walters, N. R. Conducting special events in malls. *Public Relations Journal.* November 1989, pp. 31-33.

Weatherington, R. Avoiding wrongful discharge suits. *Cardiology Management.* 1(3):14-21, 1987.

Weber, D. Alta Bates-Herrick Hospital implements service line management model, dismantles traditional nursing department. *Healthcare Organization Report.* 1(1):1-12, 1988.

Weinstein, A. Radiology Benchmarking. *Decisions in Imaging Economics.* Winter 1992.

Wilbanks, J. and Mori, K. "Quality Management: Radiology's Challenge." *Administrative Radiology.* 9(10):50-54, 1990.

Wilson, C. N. and Benn, S. A. The medicare catastrophic coverage act of 88: effects on radiology services. *Applied Radiology.* 18(3):19-22, 1989.

Wolff, G. Nonionic agents: okay they're safer—now what? *Administrative Radiology.* 9(11):92-106, 1990.

"Working with Consultants." *Healthcare Dynamics.* 1(6):1990.

Wortley, D. W. and Payne, G. R. Understanding the medicare cost report. *Health Administration Today.* 1(1):23-27, 1988.

Wright, M.L. "Communicating Through Codes." *AHRA Radiology Reimbursement Reference: To Guide You Through the Maze of Radiology Reimbursement.* AHRA. Sudbury, MA, 1991.

Zampetti, J. Predesign facilities for change. *Healthcare Strategic Management.* 8(4):12-14, 1990.

Zampetti, J. The plan to expand. *Administrative Radiology.* 9(10):65-67, 1990.

Zelch, J. V. Educated referral based leads to successful MRI practice. *MRI Quarterly.* Fall 1991.

INDEX—VOLUME 1

A

ACR Mammography Accreditation
    Program 177
ADA 22
Administrators Guide to MR 213
Advanced Video Products 135
Advancement 74
Advancement Program 75
Advancement Programs in the Workplace
    73
AIDS 16
American Cancer Society 171
American College of Radiology 121
American Healthcare Radiology Adminis-
    trators 14
American Hospital Association Demand
    Forecast Mode 205
Americans with Disabilities Act 22
angioplasty 195–196
    devices 196
        cutting devices 196
        dilatation 196
        stents 196
    percutaneous atherectomy 196
appraisal interview 61
Argon 167
Armbruster, Ben 160
AT&T/Phillips 135
autonomy 91

B

Bartolazzi, Pete 143, 145, 146
bit 125
bone densitometry 189–191
breast self-examination (BSE) 171
Brody, Dr. William R. 134
Buckley Amendment 43
bus 125
Buyers Guide to Evaluating MR Systems
    212
byte 125

C

California Medical Association 79

Canadian Workload Measurement System
    79
carbon dioxide 168
career planning 94–100
    employment interview 97
    job search 95
    resumes 95–97
Certificate of Need (CON) 149
CFO 183
Chemical Hazard Communication Standard
    216
chronological resume 96
chronological resume, sample 97
Civil Rights Act (1964) 28, 36, 38
clinical ladders 68–77
    benefits 74
    defined 68
Clinical Ladders—Question and Answers
    69
coherence 168
College of American Pathologists 79
Color Flow Mapping Doppler 157
computer networks 109
conceptual skills 6
counseling sequence
    ten steps of 64
CPT codes 152
CPU 125
criteria based 21
Criteria for Selecting a Contract Service
    Provider 107
criteria of evaluation 59
criteria-based job descriptions 24
CT 114
customer relations 100–103
    consumerism 102–103
    performance appraisal process 102
cyclotron 155

D

data compression 130
Data for Job Evaluation Process 30
Dictionary of Occupational Titles and Job
    Descript 20
Digital Radiography 157

Directory of Technologist Education in MRI
    208
Discrimination 45
display 125
Distrust Cycle 66
Dohms, James 216
Dotter, M.D., Charles 195
Dual Energy Radiography (DER) 190
Dual-Photon Absorptiometry (DPA) 190
DuPont 135

E

Economic Recovery Act (1981) 139
Employee Performance Deterioration 65
employee turnover 48
Equal Employment Opportunity Commis-
    sion 22
Equal Opportunity Act (1972) 36
Equal Pay Act (1963) 28, 38
equipment 138–148
    acquisition of 138–139
    hospitals 184
    preparing performance specifications
        140–141
    prepurchase considerations 139–
        140, 141–143
    specifications and performance stan-
        dards 140
essential functions of the job 23
Essential Job Functions 35

F

Fair Labor Standards Act (1938) 28, 38
Federal Fair Employment Practice
    Committee 39
Federal Food, Drug, and Cosmetic Act 217
financing new technology 200–204
    costs of new technology 204
    revenue variables 201
        market demand 201
        reimbursement 201
floppy disk 125
Food and Drug Administration (FDA) 152
formal retention program 91
FTEs 75

G

Gail Nielsen 73
General Electric Medical Systems 135, 212

Genesys 135
Glossary of PACS
    Terminology 136
Glossary of PET Terms 162
Gould, M.D., K. Lance 160
Gruntzig, M.D., Andreas 195

H

hard disk 125
Hard, Rob 133
hardware 115
Harrison, Sandra 70
Harvard RVS System 79
Harvey, Donald 43
Hazard Communication Guidelines for
    Compliance 220
Hazard Communication Standard 219
Hazardous Chemicals In The Workplace
    216
hazing 47
HCFA 154
Herzberg, Frederick 56
Herzberg's Motivation Maintenance Model
    58
HIV 22
How to Interview Your Future Boss 99
Human Resources (HR) Department 85

I

ICU 128
image archiving 130
Image Management and Communication
    System (IMACS) 127
image transmission 130
ineffective employee
    counseling of 62–67
    ten steps 64
infrared imaging 195

J

Jackson Memorial Hospital 135
JCAHO Recommended Plant/Safety
    Orientation 52
job analysis 37–38
    personnel functions
        compensation 38
        evaluation 38
        job descriptions 38
        job design 38

job specifications 38
   recruitment 38
   safety 38
   selection 38
   training 38
three basic steps 37
job congruence 19
job description review 26
job descriptions 17–36
job enrichment
   elements of 27
   goals of 27–28
job specification reference tool 44
job summary 21

K

Kuber, Michael S. 2
Kurzweil Applied Intelligence, Inc. 198

L

lasers 167, 167–170
   percutaneous laser angioplasty 169–170
   principle clinical uses 169
   types of 168
      Argon 168
      carbon dioxide 168
Levels of Responsibility for a Technical
   Position 76
Linc Group, Inc. 183

M

MAB agent 199
Magnetic Resonance Institute 136
Magnetic Source Imaging (MSI) 191–194
mammography 170–182
   accreditation 177–178
   customer orientation 173
   informational orgainizations 176–177
      American Cnacer Society 176
      American College of Radiology 176
      Cancer Information Service 177
      National Association of Women's
         Health Professiona 176
      National Cancer Institute 176
      Women's Healthcare Consultants 176
   physician referral or self referral 172–173
   screening centers
      proforma income statement 174
      proforma operating assumptions 175

screening mammography 171
Mammography Facility Checklist 182
Mammography Quality Standards Act of
   1992 181
manpower shortage 14–17, 16
market demand 201
Maslow, A.H. 56
Maslow's Hierarchy of Needs 56, 57
Material Safety Data Sheets (MSDA) 52
medical staff
   communication with 108–111
   improving relations 108–109
   physician bonding 109–110
memory 125
microprocessor 126
Milwaukee County Medical Complex 135
mobile technology 148–153
   acquisition costs 150–151
   advantages and disadvantages 149–150
   cardiac catheterization 153
   computed tomography 153
   lithotripsy 153
   magnetic resonance imaging 152
   mammography 153
      proforma mobile mammography 202
   reimbursement issues 151–152
modem 126
monochromatic 168
monoclonal antibodies (MABS) 199
mouse 126
MRI 114, 157, 204–212
   feasibility study 204
   financial feasibility 207
   predicting utilization 205–206
MSDS 216
Multicompetent 75
Multicredentialed 75
multidisciplinary clinical ladder program
   70

N

National Cancer Institute 172
National Electronics Manufacturers
   Association 121
NEMA-ACR 121
new employee check-in 55
new employee orientation 47–54
   appraisal interview 61
   equipment user training documentation
      54

evaluation worksheet 60
introducing 50
measuring individual's performance 60
performance appraisal 58
plant technology and safety 52
purpose of 47–49
supervisor, needs to know 49–51
North Carolina Baptist/Bowman Gray
     School of Medic 135
nuclear medicine 14, 15

O

ombudsman 108
OSHA 216
outreach 109

P

Pay grades 75
Peer Review 75
performance appraisal 58
     process 59–61
     purpose of 58–59
personnel selection process 37
PET as a Current Clinical Tool 156
PET scanners 114
physician liaison officer 108
Picture Archival Communication Systems
     (PACS) 120–126, 127
     architecture 129
     archiving 136
     coaxial cable 136
     components 129
          computed radiography 129
          in-house film distribution system 129
          optical archive system 129
          radiology information system 129
          teleradiology 129
     Computed Tomography (CT) 136
     digital 136
     digital radiography 136
     digitizer 136
     electronic network 127
     Hospital Information System (HIS) 136
     image acquisition device 136
     image processing 137
     information management system 137
     jukebox 137

leveling 137
     Magnetic Resonance (MR) 137
     modality 137
     National Electical Manufacturers
          Association (NEMA 137
     optical disk 137
     pros and cons 131–132
     Radiology Information System (RIS) 137
     viewing station 137
     windowing 137
     worksation 137
Pitt County Memorial Hospital (PCMH) 70
planning a PET facility 161
Portsman, M.D., W. 195
Position Description Development Guide
     for Diagnostic Imaging 21
Position Questionnaire 30
Positron Emission Tomography (PET) 154–
     167
     clinical applications 155–157
PPS reimbursement system 16
Privacy Act (1974) 43
productivity
     people 81–85
     relative value 79–80
     standardizing work load 78–79
     work measurement 81
professional development 91
Professional Practice Standards 73

Q

Quality Assurance 75
Quality Assurance in Mammography 178
Quality Control 75
Quality Improvement 75
quality of work life 84
Quantitative CT (QCT) 190–191

R

Radiation Control for Health and Safety Act
     (PC 90) 138
radiation therapy 14, 15
radiographers 14
radiography 15
radiologic administration 2–13
     functions of management 6–13
          controlling 6, 10–11

leading 6, 11–12
 organizing 6, 9–10
 planning 6, 7–9
 staffing 6, 12–13
radiologic technologist 14
Radiology Information Systems (RIS) 114–126
 evaluating 118
 implementing 119
 planning RIS evaluations 117
 selecting 116–117
RADWORKS 79
RAM 126
reasonable accommodation 23
recruiting and retaining staff
 retention 89–90
 aids to 90–92
 sources 86–87
 media advertisements 86
 recruiters 86
 special events 86
 strategies 87
reference letter, sample 45
references
 giving 44
 validity 43–44
Regional Medical Center 136
Registry 75
reimbursement 201
reimbursement questions 152
Relative Value Units (RVU) 79, 82
Request for Proposal (RFP) 103
 award criteria 106
retention program 101
retention strategies 17
Right-to-Know Laws 221
RIS Checklist 126
ROM 126
rubidium-82 155

S

Sample Hazard Communication Program 222
Schwartz, Howard W. 132, 207
Scripps Clinic in LaJolla 194
selection interview 39
 steps in 39–42

Shock Wave Lithotripsy 157
Siemens 136, 160
Single-Photon Absorptiometry (SPA) 190
slip ring 199
software 115
 functions of the system 115
software vendors 114
sonographers 14, 15
Specialties 75
SPECT 114
SPECT thallium 158
SQUIDS 191
Steps to Accommodating Disabled Employees 36
stroke 194
Summit on Manpower 14

T

Team Process 75
Technical Clinical Ladder 72
technology assessment 182–188
 equipment at hospitals 184
 information resources 187–191
 American Hospital Association 187
 American Medical Association 188
 Council on Health Care Technology 188
 ECRI 188
 Johns Hopkins Program for Medical Technology and P 188
 MD Buyline 188
 Medical Technology and Practice Patterns Institute 188
 National Center for Health Services Research and H 188
 planning considerations 187
teleradiology 130
Texas Instruments Company 48
TIA 194
train-the-trainer 105
trigger words 198
turf battles 170
Turnover 75

U

undue hardship 46
United States Department of Labor 21

University of Michigan Medical Center 92
University of Texas Medical School 160
University of Virginia 135

V

Verifying references 44
vertical loading 27
Veterans Administration Hospital 135
voice recognition technology 197–199
   CPT-4 199
   ICD-9 199
   trigger words 198
Vortech Data 136

W

wait states 126
What You Can and Can't Ask During an
    Interview 40
workstations 131

Y

Yag 168

INDEX—VOLUME 2

A

accreditation 174
Accreditation Manual for Hospitals 162, 187
accreditation survey 174
accumulative double apportionment 220
ACR communication guidelines 203
ADA affect the design and construction 100
admitting diagnosis 231
Agenda for Change 161
Albert Einstein Medical Center 140
Albrecht, Karl 137
American College of Surgeons 159
American Medical Association 216
American Registry of Radiologic Technologists (ARR) 150
ancillary services 231
appeals 232
appropriateness of care 263
architect 81
Architectural Process in Medical Terms 102
aspects of care, important 175
assignment 232
assignment under Medicare rules 232
Attributes of a Hassle-free Hospital 124
average length of stay (ALOS) 232

B

balance billings 232
base year costs 233
basic healthcare financial management 208–244
  budgeting basics 223–226
    capital budget 225
    cash budget 225
    final budget 225–226
    operating budget 224–225
  communicating through codes 211–219
    Diagnosis-Related Grouping (DRG) 213
    HCPCS 219–224
    ICD-9-CM 211
    procedure coding—CPT-4 215

  reimbursement lingo 212
  cost finding 219–221
  financial terms 227–245
  medicare cost report 222
  reimbursement terms 231–244
  voluntary not-for-profit hospitals 209–211
Benchmarking Steps 127
Bernard, Jack A. 257
Bittle, Lois 254
Blue Cross 210
Blue Cross and Blue Shield 233
breach of duty 190
Budget 227
business plans 7–11
  competition 9
  executive summary 7–8
  market analysis 9

C

Canadian Council on Hospital Accreditation 159
capital-related costs 233
cardiopulmonary resuscitation (CPR) 175
carriers 233
case 233
case mix 233, 263
case mix index 233
Certificate of Need (CON) 2–6
CHAMPUS 234
charges 234, 263
  actual 234
  allowable 234
clinical privileges 175
clinician-to-manager 120
CME credit 16
co-insurance 234
Collins, Dale 78
commercial insurance 210, 234
Committee on Drugs and Contrast Media of the Ameri 198
comorbidity 234, 263
compliance 175
complication 234

conformance to customer expectations 124
consultants 12–14
    choosing 13–28
    in-house 13
continuing education 175
continuity of care 263
continuous improvement 124
continuous quality improvement 263
contractual adjustment/allowance 210
contractual model 153
contrast media
    current criteria for use 201
contrast reaction lawsuits 195
controllable cost 227
Cosby, Philip B. 244
cost accounting 227
cost allocation 228
cost apportionment 228
cost center 228
cost containment 143–149
    consultant's role 144–146
    cost/benefit analysis 146–148
    eliminating programs and services 146
        exit strategy criteria 147
        profit margins for healthcare pro-
            grams 147
    financial repositioning 144
    types of benefits 148–149
        tangible economic benefits 148
cost-to-charge ratio 228
cost/benefit study 146
costs 234
    allowable 234
coverage 234
CPT-4 216, 216–217, 234
    code assignment 216
        illustration of how to use 217
credentialing 176
criteria 176
Crosby, Phillip 124
customer satisfaction 126

D

Darling v. Charleston Community
    Memorial Hospital 188
data base 263
data element 263
data trend 263
deductible 235
Deming, W. Edwards 124

Fourteen Points of 130
Department of Health and Human Services
    (HHS) 152
deposition subpoena 190
deposition subpoena duces tecum 190
Design Flaws in Planning a new MRI
    Facility 84
Diagnosis-Related Grouping (DRG)
    213, 228, 235
    circulatory system: surgical partitioning
        214
    DRG assignment 213
    payment rates 213
    principal diagnosis impact on payment
        215
diagnostic radiology services 176
differential cost 228
direct labor 228
direct material 228
direct medical education costs 235
discharge 228, 235
discharge status 235
discovery subpoenas 190
doctrine of caveat emptor 189
doctrine of respondeat superior 188
double apportionment method 220
DRG coordinator 236
DRG cost weights 235
DRG creep 236
DRG rate 236
DRG weight 228
DRGs 468, 469, 470 235

E

effectiveness of care 263
efficacy of care 264
efficiency of care 264
emergency preparedness plan/program 176
equipment management 176
excluded providers 236
expert 264
explanation of medicare benefits (EOMB)
    236

F

Facilitator Selection Criteria 131
facility planning 80–104
    conceptual design models 96–100
        freestanding 96
        hospital-attached 97

hospital-integrated 99–100
  medical mall 96
construction planning 80–84
designing for maximum workflow 86–89
  central-core design 89
  mirror-design 89
  radiographer activity circular path 87
  radiographer activity flow chart 87
  single-corridor design 86
  two-corridor design 86
  wing design 89
planning for efficient work flow 89–94
  darkrooms 93
  environment 94
  film reading 94
  fluoroscopic design 93
  records management 92
radiology procedure room sizes 95
support space 84–85
FAX 15
federal employee program (FEP) 236
federal rate 236
fee for service 228
final diagnosis 237
financial innovations 146
financial revitalization 144
fiscal intermediary (FI) 237
fixed costs 220, 228
focused preparation process 164
FTEs per occupied bed 221
full costs 229
function 264
fundamental quality improvement
  philosophy 126

G

general ledger 229
general plant and technology safety 167
global fee 237
Glossary of CQI Terms 263
Glossary of Financial Terms 227
Glossary of JCAHO Terms 174
Glossary of Reimbursement Terms 231
Goodhart, Mark 140
gross margin 229
Grouper 214, 229, 237
guideline, scoring 177

H

HCPCS 219, 237

billing information 219
reasons for incorrect radiology reimbursement 220
UB-82 219
Health Care Financing Administration
  (HCFA) 213, 237
health care organization 264
Health Insurance Manual 15 (HIM15) 222
HHS safe harbor regulations 154
high-risk function 264
high-volume function 264
historical-continuous expense budgeting
  223
HMO 237
hospital economic factors 221
  bad debt 221
  cash flow 221
  depreciation 221
  interest 221
hospital-specific rate 238
Hunton, Bud W. 82

I

ICD-9-CM
  base code 211
  E code 213
  V code 213
ICD9-CM 238
In Search of Excellence 25
incremental cost 228
indication 264
indicator 264
indicator rationale 264
indicator statement 264
indirect medical education costs 238
industrial workers compensation plans 238
informed consent 195
Initiating an Improvement Project 135
integrated cost accounting 220
intent of standard 177
internal service 137
investment model 154

J

Jaffe, Dennis 145
JCAHO Recommended Plant/Safety
  Orientation 65
Johns Hopkins Hospital 15
Joint Commission on Accreditation of H
  159–186, 177

development of standards 161–163
glossary of JCAHO terms 174–179
implementation of standards 163
pre-JCAHO survey tips 172
preparing for site visits 164–166
mock survey 166
purpose of 160–161
scoring guidelines 164
survey interview 171
joint ventures 152–159
financial concerns 158
forms of 153–154
HHS safe harbor regulations 154–156
"60-40" rules 155
grandfathering 156
space and equipment rental 156
managing the joint venture process 157–158
operational issues 158
Juran, J.P. 124

K

key function 264
Kubler-Ross, Elizabeth 145

L

licensed independent practitioner 177
licensure of radiologic professionals 149–152
limited licensure 150–151
nuclear medicine 151
radiation therapy 151
radiography 151
states with licensure laws 150
Life Safety Inspection 179

M

Major diagnosis 229
major diagnosis 229
major diagnostic category (MDC) 229, 238
malpractice suit 189
managed care 210
management by exception 229
Managing Successful Radiology Projects 85
marginal cost 229
marketing imaging services 16–34
narrow view perspective 16–21
accessibility 19
consumer information 17

pricing 19
product development 18
strategic planning 18
McDonald restaurant 82
mean 265
MECON Associates, San Ramon, Calif 138
medicaid 210, 238
medical record 229
medical record review 265
medical review entities 238
medical specialty 229
medical staff 177
medically unnecessary services and custodial care 239
medicare 209, 229, 239
part A 209, 230
part B 209, 230
Medicare and Medicaid Anti-kickback Statute 154
Medicare and Medicaid Patient and Program Protecti 152
medicare code editor 214
Medicare Prospective Payment System (PPS) 213
Medicare/Medicaid Anti-Fraud and Abuse Statute 154
Medicare/Medicaid Patient and Program Protection A 158
medigap 239
mission statement 177
monitoring and evaluation 178
Mori, M.D., Kurt 245

N

National Health Planning and Resources Development 2
new managers 120–123
habits of effective managers 122–123
creativity 123
independence 122
listening skills 122
negotiation skills 123
self-discipline 122
teamwork 123
understanding 123
leading management styles 122
authoritative managers 122
coach managers 122
coercive managers 122
democratic managers 122

pacesetting managers 122
management style 121–122
management training 121
strategies for being successful 123–124
success as a new supervisor 121
nonaccumulative double apportionment
220
Nowak, Stephen F. 226
nuclear medicine services 178

O

operating margin 229
operating room (OR) procedure 239
"OR" procedure hierarchy 239
organization unit 265
orientation, training and education of staff
members 170
other diagnoses 239
other procedures 240
outcome 265
outliers 240
overhead 229

P

participating physicians 240
pass-through costs 240
patient anxiety 192
patient billing 230
Patient, family education 169
Patient Satisfaction Survey 31
PET scanners 15
Peters, Tom 25
phases of change 145
Physician Satisfaction Survey 29
ping-ponging 240
planning suggestions 103–104
policies and procedures 59–68
auditing 67
benefits of 63–64
JCAHO review 64–65
policy management 60, 62
policy statements 62
preparing the manual 64
check points 64
orgainizing 65–67
Pratt v. Davis 194
pre-admission testing 240
preferred provider organization (PPO)
230, 240
Premier Hospitals Alliance 138

price variance 230
prime cost 230
principal diagnosis 240
principal procedure 240
process indicator 265
product cost 230
product costing 230
product line 230
professional component 241
professional review organization (PRO)
241
prospective payment 230, 241
Prospective payment assessment commission 241
provider 265
proximate cause 190
Public Law 89-97 (Medicare) 160

Q

quality assessment 178
quality assessment and improvement
168, 178, 244–266
aspects of care 253–254
indicator development 254–266
JCAHO's Ten-Step Process 247–250
quality assessment and improvement
plan (example) 250–253
quality improvement process 245–246
quality improvement 178
quality improvement group 128
quality of patient care 265
quantity variance 231
Questionnaires and Interviews 30

R

radiation oncology services 178
radiologic organizations 35
radiology codes 216
radiology procedures 101–102
rate per diem 231
rate variance 230
referral centers 241
regional rate 241
reimbursement 241
cost-based 231, 242
prospective 242
retrospective 242
relative value unit (RVU) 231
reliability assessment 265
Repeat Referral Business to MRI 22

responsibility accounting 231
risk management and liability prevention
    187–208
  activities 187
  court subpoenas 190–191
  informed consent 194–197
    in radiology 195–197
  legal environment 188–190
    equipment-related malpractice claims
      189
    hospital duties 189
    malpractice suits 189
  liability prevention checklist 192–194

S

Safety Profiles 180
scope of care 265
Scoring Guidelines 162
Scott, Cynthia 145
self-pay insurance 210
sentinel event 266
service line management 118–120
  imaging 119–121
service line management benefits 118
service line thinking 118
Social Security Act 154
Social Security Amendments of 1965 (Title
  XVIII) 209
soft areas 85
sole community hospitals 242
Special Policy on Safety 184
St. Paul Insurance Company 188
standard 178, 266
standard cost 231
standard of care 189
standards-based quality-of-care evaluation
  266
step-down method 220
Stereotactic Breast Biopsy 218
strategic planning 68–79
  defined 72–73
  mission statement 69
  process 73
    steps in 73–78
  setting department goals 74–75
Strauch, Dan 140
supplementary medical insurance 209

T

technical component 242
TEFRA 242
third-party 243
threshold 266
timeliness of care 266
Top 10 Service Strategies for Boosting
  Referrals 22
total quality management 124–138
  measuring seccess 132–144
  principles for sound quality effort 128–
    131
  problem-solving steps 128
  quaility vision 126
  quality self-assessment survey 131–132
traffic patterns 86
transfer 242
trial subpoena 191
Trout, M. D., Monroe E. 257
Type I recommendation 179
Type II recommendation 179

U

unbundling 243
uniform bill-payment summary (UB-82)
  219, 243
uniform institutional provider bill 219
updating factor 243
utilization management 243
utilization statistic 231

V

validity assessment 266
variable cost 231
variance 231

W

wage index 243
Weinstein, Alan 138
Westrend Group 131
Wietmarschen, George A. 141
Wilbanks, John 245
World Health Organization Center for
  Classificatio 211
written informed consent procedure 196
  sample 197

Y

Yale University 213

Z

Zampetti, James 82
Zerhouni, MD., Elias 15
zero-based 223

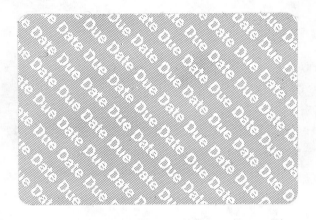